DR. SEBI MUCUS CLEANSE BIBLE

The Definitive Guide to Quickly Remove Excess Mucus and Deep Cleanse Your Body with Dr. Sebi Recommended Herbs and Foods | 28-Day Detox Plan Included

Valeria-Cruz Mendez

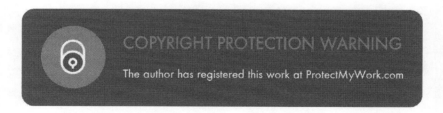

Table of Contents

INTRODUCTION

Welcome, dear reader. *"Dr. Sebi Mucus Cleanse Bible"* is to guide you through understanding and applying Dr. Sebi's profound teachings to optimize your health by removing excess mucus from your body.

For those unfamiliar, Dr. Sebi was a renowned herbalist and healer whose approach to wellness centers on nutrition and natural remedies. His philosophy emphasizes the importance of an alkaline diet and the detoxification process, turning our focus towards plant-based foods and herbal solutions.

Mucus, though a normal body substance that plays protective roles, can become problematic when produced in excess. It starts clogging our systems, impairing our bodily functions, and contributing to various health issues. This book will help you grasp the significance of mucus management for overall wellness.

We start by exploring Dr. Sebi's health principles and why detoxification is key. You'll learn how excess mucus can negatively affect your respiratory system, digestive health, and even lead to chronic diseases like sinusitis or bronchitis. Through the real-life stories of people like Susan and Mark, you'll see the impact of unresolved mucus issues and how cleansing can bring relief.

Next, we'll discuss the methodology behind Dr. Sebi's mucus cleanse—understanding why certain herbs and foods are effective in mucus removal. With scientific backing interwoven with traditional wisdom, you'll be given clear guidelines on how to use liver-, kidney-, lung-, and skin-cleaning herbs.

Preparing for a cleanse is crucial for success, so I'll provide practical steps to get you ready both mentally and physically for this journey. We'll tackle common fears, set realistic expectations, and outline how to transition smoothly into a plant-based diet that's vigorous enough to support your cleansing goals.

The heart of this book lies in the 28-day detox plan designed by Dr. Sebi himself. You'll find a week-by-week guide starting from transitioning phases to deep cleansing, fasting resets, and finishing with reintroduction strategies to maintain your newfound health benefits long-term.

Additionally, I'll share numerous recipes meticulously tailored for breakfast, lunch, dinner, and snacks—each one compliant with Dr. Sebi's recommendations. These recipes not only promise nourishment but also support your detox pathway ensuring an enjoyable experience throughout your cleanse.

Incorporating these principles into daily life might seem daunting at first; hence the book includes practical advice on sustaining these lifestyle changes amidst everyday routines including dining out or traveling. Whether you're doing it solo or adapting it for family members' needs—including children or the elderly—you'll find helpful tips here.

And let's face it: challenges will arise during any major lifestyle overhaul. That's why I've dedicated a section to overcoming these obstacles using pragmatic solutions you can easily incorporate into your routine while keeping long-term health improvements in focus.

To enhance you further post-cleanse experience there's a chapter on maintaining these changes long beyond the initial 28 days with advanced detox strategies seamlessly aligned with Dr. Sebi's teachings.

Lastly comes an extensive FAQ section addressing common queries about herbal supplements dietary adjustments along clarifying misconceptions about the alkaline diet helping you embark on this journey more informed confident than ever before concluding our exploration with final thoughts on holistic healing inviting healthier way living natural way!

Dr. Sebi's Philosophy and Holistic Health Principles

Dr. Sebi, born Alfredo Bowman, was a Honduran herbalist who believed that a return to natural foods was key for optimal health. His philosophy is centered around the concept of an alkaline diet and herbal remedies. Essentially, he argued that our modern diet is filled with acidic foods that contribute to mucus buildup in our bodies, leading to various diseases.

One of Dr. Sebi's primary principles is the idea that disease stems from an acidic environment within the body. He believed that by adopting an alkaline diet—one high in plant-based foods—we can restore our body to a state of health. The principle here is simple: disease cannot survive in an alkaline environment.

So, what exactly constitutes an alkaline diet? It's primarily composed of natural, raw fruits and vegetables, along with certain grains, seeds, nuts, and oils. Here is a brief guide:

ALKALINE FOODS	ACIDIC FOODS TO AVOID
Leafy greens	Meat
Fruits	Dairy
Vegetables	Processed foods
Nuts	Sugar

Dr. Sebi also emphasized the importance of removing mucus from the body. According to him, excess mucus forms as a result of consuming acidic foods and creates an ideal environment for diseases like diabetes, hypertension, and other chronic conditions. He prescribed using specific herbs known for their cleansing properties to help remove this excess mucus.

The herbal remedies promoted by Dr. Sebi come from his research into indigenous herbs from Africa and the Americas. They are selected based on their ability to cleanse the body's cells at the intracellular level. Some prominent herbs in his teachings include burdock root, sarsaparilla root, and dandelion.

Another important aspect of Dr. Sebi's philosophy involves fasting or detoxifying the body periodically to remove toxins accumulated over time due to unhealthy eating habits and environmental factors. His 28-Day Detox Plan is widely recognized for significantly improving overall health by thoroughly cleansing the blood and digestive system.

Dr. Sebi also advocated against synthetic medications and processed supplements. He argued that nature provides all necessary nutrients through food and herbs when they are consumed in their most natural state.

CORE PRINCIPLE	EXPLANATION
Alkaline Diet	Consuming plant-based foods (fruits, vegetables) to keep body's pH level in an alkaline state
Mucus Removal	Using herbs to cleanse excess mucus caused by acidic foods
Herbal Remedies	Relying on natural herbs for cell-level cleansing and healing
Periodic Fasting/Detox	Detoxifying body regularly to remove accumulated toxins

Avoidance of Synthetic Substances	Reliance on natural foods over synthetic drugs or supplements

It's clear that Dr. Sebi's approach centers around simplicity and returning to nature for health solutions. By following an alkaline diet rich in whole foods, using cleansing herbs, avoiding processed products, and periodically fasting or detoxifying our bodies, we can find a path toward better health.

As you proceed through this book, remember these foundational principles of Dr. Sebi's philosophy—they're not just about mitigating symptoms but aiming for holistic wellness by addressing root causes.

Importance of Mucus Removal and Detoxification for Overall Health

Mucus is a thick, slippery substance that lines various parts of our body such as the respiratory tract, digestive tract, and reproductive organs. Its primary purpose is to protect these areas by trapping foreign particles such as dust, bacteria, and viruses. So yes, mucus serves as a critical defense mechanism for the body. However, when our body produces too much mucus or when this mucus becomes thick and sticky, it can cause several health issues. Accumulation of excess mucus can obstruct normal functions in the body. For instance, thickened mucus can block airways leading to difficulty in breathing or chronic respiratory conditions like asthma or bronchitis.

Here's where detoxification comes into play. Detoxification is the body's natural process of removing toxins that accumulate over time from various sources such as food, pollution, and even stress. When we talk about detoxification concerning mucus removal, we're specifically focusing on cleaning out excess mucus from the body to restore its normal functioning.

So why exactly do we need to remove excess mucus from our bodies? Here are some critical reasons:

1. **Breathing Easier:** Excessive mucus in the respiratory system can make it difficult to breathe comfortably. By removing this excess mucus, we can improve our lung function and ensure better oxygen exchange.

2. **Improved Digestion:** Mucus build-up in the intestines can hamper nutrient absorption and lead to bloating or digestive discomforts. Clearing out this excess helps improve digestion and nutrient assimilation.

3. **Reducing Infections:** Stagnant mucus can become a breeding ground for bacteria and viruses. By maintaining regular mucus removal through detoxification practices, we reduce the risk of infections.

4. **Increasing Energy Levels:** When your body isn't overloaded with excessive toxins or struggling with blocked systems due to mucus build-up, you naturally feel more energetic.

Let's look at how we can effectively eliminate excess mucus from the body:

1. **Hydration:** Drinking plenty of water is fundamental to thinning out thickened mucus so that it can be easily expelled from the body.

2. **Herbal Teas:** Certain herbal teas like ginger tea or peppermint tea have been known to help break down excess mucus.

3. **Steaming**: Inhaling steam loosens nasal congestion by moistening your respiratory tract.

4. **Proper Diet:** Avoiding foods that stimulate excessive mucus production like dairy products and instead consuming anti-inflammatory foods such as fruits, vegetables high in Vitamin C (like oranges), and leafy greens helps manage healthy mucus levels.

5. **Regular Exercise:** This promotes respiratory health by helping clear out any congestion through deep breaths which facilitates removal of trapped particles or excessive secretions within lungs.

Incorporating these simple habits into your daily routine significantly supports your body's natural detoxification processes keeping your systems clean-balanced implying healthier lungs-digestive tracts amongst others ensuring optimal wellness generally!

CHAPTER 1

Mucus and Its Impact on Health

Mucus is that slippery, gooey stuff your body makes. It might not be the most glamorous thing to talk about, but it plays a huge role in keeping us healthy. You can think of mucus as your body's natural defense layer. It's produced by mucous membranes which line many parts of our bodies like the nose, throat, sinuses, and lungs.

So why do we even have mucus? Why does our body bother producing this sticky substance? The simple answer: protection. Here's how it works:

1. **Moistening Air Passages:** Every time you inhale, your mucus ensures that the airways in your lungs are moist. Dry air can damage these delicate passages but thanks to mucus, they remain supple and can function properly.

2. **Trapping Debris:** Imagine all the dust, pollen, germs, and dirt particles floating around us. Without mucus acting as a barrier, these foreign invaders would easily enter our body through our respiratory system. Mucus traps these unwanted particles so they can be expelled from our bodies through coughing or sneezing.

3. **Fighting Infections:** Mucus contains antibodies and enzymes that actively fight off pathogens. Those harmful bacteria and viruses that we encounter daily are no match for the defensive properties found within our mucus.

4. **Lubrication:** Mucus also helps to keep things moving smoothly inside us! It lines our digestive tract to make sure food slides effortlessly through the gut without causing damage or irritation to the lining of our intestines.

Now that we've established why mucus is so important, let's look at what makes our bodies produce it. Several factors can trigger mucus production:

1. **Infections:** When you're coming down with a cold or the flu, your body ramps up mucus production to trap and expel the invading viruses or bacteria.

2. **Allergies:** When you're allergic to something like pollen or pet dander, your immune system goes into overdrive trying to protect you from what it mistakenly sees as harmful invaders. This results in more mucus being produced to trap these allergens.

3. **Irritants:** Smoke from a cigarette or pollution in the air can irritate your mucous membranes and lead to an increase in mucus.

4. **Dehydration:** Believe it or not, if you're dehydrated your body produces thicker mucus as compensation for lack of moisture elsewhere.

5. **Diet:** Some foods are known to cause excess mucus production – dairy products are often cited as culprits for many people because they can thicken mucus.

6. **Hormonal Changes:** Hormone levels can also influence mucus production – for example, many women notice increased nasal congestion during pregnancy due to hormonal shifts.

When Mucus Becomes a Health Issue

Imagine sitting on your couch with a scratchy throat, sneezing away, and constantly blowing your nose. You're surrounded by tissues and you think to yourself, *"Is my body producing an endless supply of this stuff?"* That's what it feels like when mucus production goes into overdrive. But why does this happen?

Well, our bodies produce extra mucus as a defense mechanism. If there's an invader like bacteria or viruses or even something we're allergic to, our body kicks mucus production into high gear to trap those nasty intruders and expel them from our system. Healthy mucus is clear and thin. However when our system detects trouble – such as an infection – it turns thick and discolored as it traps germs and debris.

Here's where things can get tricky: An excess of thickened mucus isn't just annoying; it can become downright problematic for our health:

1. **Respiratory Issues:** Too much mucus in your respiratory system can block your airways. This makes breathing more difficult and can even lead to infections. If you have asthma or bronchitis for instance, extra mucus can make these conditions much worse.

2. **Sinus Congestion:** Excessive nasal mucus leads to clogged sinuses. This causes pressure around your eyes and face, making you feel miserable. Sinus headaches are literally headaches caused by congestion-induced pressure.

3. **Digestive Problems:** It's not just confined to the nose and throat; excess mucus in the digestive system can cause problems like bloating and indigestion by interfering with the digestive process.

4. **Hearing Issues:** Your ears aren't safe either! When there is excessive mucus in your Eustachian tubes (the tubes that help balance pressure in your ears), this may lead to ear infections or even temporary hearing loss.

AREA	COMMON SYMPTOMS
Nose & Throat	Congestion, sore throat
Respiratory	Coughing, wheezing
Digestive System	Bloating, indigestion
Ears	Pain, temporary hearing loss

Connection Between Excess Mucus and Common Diseases

Many of us don't realize how crucial it is to maintain balance in our bodies, and mucus plays a surprisingly pivotal part. When there's too much mucus, it can lead to several health issues that are more common than you might think. Let me break this down for you.

1. **Chronic Sinusitis:** One of the most prevalent issues tied to excess mucus is chronic sinusitis. When we have too much mucus, it clogs our sinuses, causing pain, congestion, and pressure. Imagine trying to breathe through a straw—you'd feel stuffy and uncomfortable.

2. **Asthma:** Excess mucus in the airways can make breathing a real challenge for people with asthma. When there's too much mucus built up, it narrows the airways and triggers wheezing, coughing, and shortness of breath. Keeping those lungs clear of unnecessary mucus is crucial for controlling asthma symptoms.

3. **Chronic Obstructive Pulmonary Disease (COPD):** In conditions like COPD, excessive mucus production obstructs airflow, making it difficult to breathe. This buildup aggravates symptoms like persistent coughing and frequent respiratory infections. It's kind of like trying to suck a thick shake through a small straw—it takes so much effort!

4. **Bronchitis:** When we get bronchitis, our bronchial tubes get inflamed, leading to an overproduction of mucus. This results in a relentless cough that often brings up phlegm or sputum. It feels like there's always something stuck in your throat that you just can't clear out.

5. **Cystic Fibrosis:** Cystic fibrosis causes thick and sticky mucus buildup in various organs including the lungs and digestive system. This excess mucus makes it hard for sufferers to breathe and can lead to severe lung infections over time.

6. **Pneumonia:** Bacterial or viral pneumonia often comes with an enormous amount of mucus filling our lungs' air sacs. The body tries to fight off the infection by sending more mucus to the site, which unfortunately makes breathing even harder.

7. **Gastroesophageal Reflux Disease (GERD):** We usually think of GERD as causing heartburn but did you know it can also lead to excess mucus? That irritating acid reflux can result in a feeling of chronic postnasal drip or throat clearing as your body tries to manage the irritation.

8. **Ear Infections:** You might not immediately connect your ears with mucus, but it's all related! When you have more than normal nasal discharge due to allergies or colds, it can travel up into the Eustachian tubes in your ears, leading to painful ear infections.

9. **Sleep Apnea:** Excess nasal and throat mucus can weigh down soft tissues while you sleep, obstructing airflow and causing obstructive sleep apnea.

10. **Allergic Rhinitis (Hay Fever):** This common allergy produces tons of extra mucus as your body reacts to pollen or dust mites with sneezing and runny nose—definitely not fun during allergy season!

11. **High Blood Pressure:** Believe it or not, excess mucus can also be a hidden contributor to high blood pressure. When our bodies are trying to pump through all that extra congestion, it can lead to increased strain on our cardiovascular system. This might sound surprising, but managing your mucus levels can actually help keep your blood pressure in check.

12. **Diabetes:** Excess mucus can also impact people with diabetes in unexpected ways. High blood sugar levels can lead to more mucus production. This can create a vicious cycle where the body's efforts to manage glucose levels end up causing more congestion and related issues.

COMMON DISEASE	CONNECTION WITH EXCESS MUCUS
Chronic Sinusitis	Excess mucus clogs sinuses, causing pain and congestion.
Asthma	Mucus narrows airways, triggering wheezing and shortness of breath.
Chronic Obstructive Pulmonary Disease (COPD)	Mucus obstructs airflow, making breathing difficult.
Bronchitis	Inflammation causes overproduction of mucus, leading to relentless cough.
Cystic Fibrosis	Thick mucus buildup makes breathing hard and causes lung infections.

Pneumonia	Infection leads to excess mucus filling lung air sacs, making breathing harder.
Gastroesophageal Reflux Disease (GERD)	Acid reflux causes postnasal drip or throat clearing due to irritation-managed by extra mucus.
Ear Infections	Excess nasal discharge travels up Eustachian tubes, leading to painful infections.
Sleep Apnea	Nasal and throat mucus obstructs airflow during sleep, causing OSA (Obstructive Sleep Apnea).
Allergic Rhinitis (Hay Fever)	Allergic reactions produce tons of extra mucus as response to allergens like pollen or dust mites, causing sneezing
High Blood Pressure	Excess mucus increases cardiovascular strain by forcing the body to pump through the congestion.
Diabetes	High blood sugar levels cause more mucus production, creating additional health complications for diabetics.

By understanding these connections better we may make more informed choices regarding diet lifestyle ultimately aiming towards reducing unnecessary mucous build-up fostering overall wellness! Remember moderation key tracking how consuming feels don't hesitate tweaking habits accordingly achieving best results personalized needs respective journey healthier self!

Case Studies of the Negative Impacts of Excess Mucus

When it comes to understanding how excess mucus can affect our daily lives, nothing hits home quite like real stories from real people. Below, I'll share two case studies that illustrate just how debilitating excess mucus can be.

Case Study 1: Susan's Struggle with Chronic Sinusitis

Susan, a 34-year-old mother of two, thought her constant fatigue and frequent headaches were just part of the hectic life of being a parent. However, when the symptoms persisted despite getting rest and eating well, she knew something was wrong. She was often plagued by a stuffy nose and sinus pressure that made it difficult to focus at work or enjoy family time.

After multiple visits to various doctors, Susan was diagnosed with chronic sinusitis—a condition characterized by inflamed and swollen sinuses. Her doctor explained that excess mucus production was blocking her nasal passages, causing the persistent headaches and fatigue. Although she tried several prescription medications, they only offered temporary relief.

The turning point came when Susan decided to take matters into her own hands. She began a regimen aimed at reducing mucus naturally. This included dietary changes like cutting out dairy and processed foods, known contributors to mucus production. She also started practicing steam inhalation and nasal irrigation regularly.

Within weeks, Susan noticed a significant reduction in her symptoms. Her sinus pressure reduced, her headaches became less frequent, and she even experienced an increase in energy levels. By addressing the root cause—excess mucus—Susan reclaimed her everyday life.

Case Study 2: Mark's Battle with Chronic Bronchitis

Mark, a 50-year-old fitness enthusiast, never imagined that excess mucus could hinder his active lifestyle. Known amongst his friends as someone who rarely got sick, Mark was caught off guard when he developed a persistent cough that refused to go away.

Initially dismissing it as a common cold or seasonal allergies, he continued his daily gym workouts and running routines. But as weeks turned into months, Mark's cough worsened, accompanied by shortness of breath and wheezing attacks during exercise. Concerned about his deteriorating health, he visited his physician who diagnosed him with chronic bronchitis.

Chronic bronchitis is characterized by continuous inflammation in the bronchial tubes with an overproduction of mucus that clogs these airways. Mark was prescribed inhalers and anti-inflammatory drugs but experienced minimal relief.

Frustrated but determined not to let this condition dictate his life, Mark consulted a holistic health practitioner who advised him on several lifestyle changes focused on reducing mucus buildup. Along with quitting smoking—which he realized had aggravated his condition—Mark shifted to an alkaline diet rich in fruits and vegetables. He also included herbal teas known for their anti-inflammatory properties.

In three months' time, Mark's coughing episodes reduced drastically; he no longer experienced shortness of breath during workouts. Reinvigorated by his improved health condition, Mark became an advocate for addressing excess mucus through natural methods within his local fitness community.

Final Thoughts

These case studies highlight how excess mucus can severely impact quality of life. Whether it's interfering with daily responsibilities like in Susan's case or hampering an active lifestyle as it did for Mark, addressing the root cause of mucus production can make a world of difference.

In both situations, traditional medical treatments offered limited relief, emphasizing the importance of holistic approaches. Simple changes like diet modifications and natural remedies can significantly reduce mucus buildup and improve overall well-being. Susan cutting out dairy and processed foods, and Mark adopting an alkaline diet rich in fruits and vegetables, were pivotal in their respective recoveries.

If you're struggling with similar issues, consider exploring natural solutions to manage excess mucus. Small adjustments to your daily habits might just be the key to reclaiming your health and vitality. Remember, everyone's journey is unique, but these stories show that there is hope. You can overcome the debilitating effects of excess mucus with the right approach and mindset.

CHAPTER 2

The Science Behind Dr. Sebi's Mucus Cleanse

Overview of the Herbs and Foods Dr. Sebi Recommends for Mucus Removal

Dr. Sebi recommended an alkaline diet to minimize the accumulation of mucus in the body. His approach primarily revolved around consuming natural, plant-based foods that help maintain an alkaline pH in our systems. This type of diet aids in preventing the overproduction of mucus and supports detoxification naturally.

One of the core elements of Dr. Sebi's diet is herbs. He strongly believed in their ability to cleanse the body, promote digestion, and boost overall health without causing harmful side effects like synthetic medications might.

Let's dig into some of the key herbs and foods recommended by Dr. Sebi for mucus removal:

Herbs Recommended by Dr. Sebi

1. **Burdock Root:** Burdock root is one of Dr. Sebi's go-to herbs due to its powerful detoxifying properties. It's a blood purifier, which means it helps remove toxins from your bloodstream. By doing so, it supports almost every part of your body, especially the liver and kidneys.
2. **Sarsaparilla:** Sarsaparilla is packed with minerals like iron, which is essential for maintaining energy levels and overall vitality. This herb also has anti-inflammatory properties, making it great for reducing swelling and pain in the joints.
3. **Elderberry**: Elderberry is a fantastic immune booster, which is crucial because a strong immune system helps fend off illnesses before they get a chance to take hold. It's particularly great during cold seasons as it can help alleviate symptoms of the flu and common cold.

4. **Dandelion Root:** Dandelion root is another herb that's excellent for detoxification. It promotes healthy liver function and improves digestion by stimulating bile production. Regular use can help keep your digestive system in check and free from bloating and discomfort.

5. **Bladderwrack:** Bladderwrack is particularly famous for its high iodine content, which supports thyroid health—a critical part of regulating metabolism in our bodies. This seaweed also contains essential vitamins and minerals that make it a superb addition to a healthy diet.

6. **Yellow Dock:** Yellow dock works wonders for the digestive system as well. It has mild laxative properties that gently cleanse the gut without causing discomfort or dependency.

7. **Nettle Leaf:** Nettle leaf is rich in nutrients such as iron, calcium, magnesium, and vitamins A and K. It's known for helping with allergies and boosting overall nutrient levels in the body.

HERB NAME	MAIN BENEFITS	KEY MINERALS
Burdock Root	Blood purification	Potassium, Iron
Sarsaparilla	Anti-inflammatory & iron source	Iron
Elderberry	Immune system boost	Vitamin C, Fiber
Dandelion Root	Liver support & digestion aid	Potassium
Bladderwrack	Thyroid support	Iodine
Yellow Dock	Digestive cleansing	Calcium, Magnesium
Nettle Leaf	Nutrient-rich support	Iron, Calcium

Dr. Sebi's approach to using these herbs isn't just about taking them individually; it's about integrating them into a holistic lifestyle that promotes cleansing and nourishes the body from within.

How To Use These Herbs

1. **Teas:** One of the simplest ways to consume these herbs is through herbal teas. For instance, you can make nettle tea or dandelion root tea.

2. **Capsules:** If you're not keen on teas or tinctures, capsules are an excellent option available at most health stores.

3. **Powders:** These can be easily added to smoothies or juices.

4. **Tinctures:** Concentrated liquid extracts where you usually need only a few drops mixed with water or juice.

Foods Recommended by Dr. Sebi

1. **Green Leafy Vegetables:** Veggies like spinach, kale, and Swiss chard are alkaline-forming foods that help maintain your body's pH levels conducive to health, thereby limiting mucus production.
2. **Fruits like Berries:** Blueberries, raspberries, strawberries they're not only delicious but packed with antioxidants that help fight inflammation and reduce mucus.
3. **Avocado:** Full of healthy fats, avocados help lubricate cell membranes which aid in reducing mucus buildup.
4. **Cucumber**: High water content in cucumbers keeps you hydrated and flushes toxins out of your system, reducing excess mucus.
5. **Squash:** Especially yellow squash which contains nutrients that help in clearing out lungs' congestion.
6. **Sea Moss:** An outstanding source of minerals (it contains 92 of 102 essential minerals we need!), sea moss is exceptional for dissolving inflammation and removing excess mucus from the body.

Simple Integration Ideas

1. Start your day with a herbal tea made from burdock root or sarsaparilla.
2. Add ginger or cayenne pepper to your meals for an extra health boost.
3. Make a refreshing smoothie with a mix of berries—I love combining blueberries and strawberries!
4. Slice avocado into your salad or spread it on toast.
5. Incorporate leafy greens into soups or stews.
6. Snack on cucumber slices dipped in hummus.
7. Prepare a sea moss gel to add into shakes or use as a thickener in recipes.

Scientific or Traditional Backing for the Efficacy of These Herbs and Foods

According to various traditional and holistic approaches, including Dr. Sebi's teachings, excess mucus is linked to many health issues. Now, we look to nature's pharmacy—the amazing world of herbs and alkaline foods—to help cleanse our bodies.

1. **Burdock Root:** This herb has been used for centuries in traditional medicine. Burdock root is celebrated for its blood-purifying properties, essential for detoxifying the body. Modern research supports this, showing that it contains phenolic acids, quercetin, and luteolin — compounds known for their antioxidant and anti-inflammatory properties. These elements help detoxify the blood and support liver health by enhancing liver function, crucial for filtering toxins from the body.

2. **Sarsaparilla:** Traditionally used to treat skin conditions like psoriasis and eczema and to improve energy levels, modern scientific studies have confirmed that sarsaparilla indeed has potent anti-inflammatory and immune-boosting capabilities. Its high iron content is significant as iron plays a vital role in maintaining energy levels by aiding in oxygen transport within the bloodstream.

3. **Elderberry:** Traditional practices have long utilized this berry to boost the immune system, especially during cold seasons. Science backs this up; elderberries are rich in flavonoids, which give them their strong antioxidant properties. Various studies indicate that elderberry extract can reduce the duration and severity of cold and flu symptoms, supporting its role as an excellent immune booster.

4. **Dandelion Root:** Traditionally known for its detoxifying qualities, dandelion root stimulates bile production, aiding digestion and liver health. Contemporary scientific studies echo these findings, showing that dandelion root has diuretic properties that help in flushing out toxins from the kidneys while supporting digestive health through improved bile flow.

5. **Bladderwrack:** It's a type of seaweed, has gained recognition both traditionally and scientifically. Known primarily for its high iodine content, bladderwrack supports thyroid health which is crucial for regulating metabolism. Additionally, bladderwrack contains a variety of vitamins and minerals that bolster overall well-being.

6. **Yellow Dock:** Often flies under the radar but has been traditionally revered for its digestive benefits. It has mild laxative properties that gently cleanse the gut without causing discomfort or dependency. Scientific research reveals that yellow dock contains anthraquinones which contribute to its laxative effects and hepatoprotective properties.

7. **Nettle Leaf:** It is a powerhouse of nutrients such as iron, calcium, magnesium, and vitamins A and K. Traditional medicine has long praised nettle leaf for boosting nutrient levels and alleviating allergy symptoms. Science now validates these uses; nettle leaves contain biologically active compounds like flavonoids which have antioxidant properties that help in reducing inflammation.

Now let's talk about some of Dr. Sebi's recommended foods.

1. **Green Leafy Vegetables:** Leafy Vegetables like spinach, kale, and Swiss chard are alkaline-forming foods crucial in maintaining our body's pH levels conducive to health and limiting mucus production. Scientifically speaking, these vegetables are rich in chlorophyll—known to detoxify the blood—and fiber which aids digestion hand-in-hand with other essential nutrients needed for optimal body function.

2. **Berries:** Blueberries, raspberries, and strawberries are not only delicious but packed with antioxidants like vitamin C which fight inflammation—a key factor in reducing mucus levels within our bodies.

3. **Avocado:** This creamy delight is high in healthy fats which help lubricate cell membranes, aiding in reducing mucus buildup. Modern studies support this too – good fats keep our cells healthy and functioning optimally. Traditionally in Central American cultures where avocados originate from, they've been valued greatly not just for their taste but their health benefits too.

4. **Cucumbers:** With their high-water content, cucumbers hydrate us and flush out toxins — vital for reducing mucus. Science backs this up; hydration is key in thinning mucus and preventing congestion. Historically speaking, cucumbers were often used in ancient Ayurvedic practices in India to cool and cleanse the body.

5. **Yellow Squash:** It's packed with nutrients that benefit our lungs' health by clearing out congestion. Studies have shown it contains compounds like beta-carotene which supports respiratory function by reducing inflammation – consequently reducing mucus production. Traditionally among Native American diets, squash was a staple food revered for its multitude of health benefits.

6. **Sea Moss:** This incredible seaweed contains 92 of 102 essential minerals our body needs! Scientifically proven to dissolve inflammation effectively makes it a champion at removing excess mucus from the body system. The historical usage of sea moss traces back over millennia especially among coastal communities who knew well about its healing benefits long before scientific validation came along.

The Body's Detox Pathways: Liver, Kidneys, Lungs, and Skin

Knowing about the body's detox pathways is crucial for maintaining good health. Our bodies are constantly exposed to toxins from the environment, food, and even internally generated waste products. Understanding the mechanisms our bodies use to rid themselves of these harmful substances is essential not only for health professionals but also for anyone looking to optimize their well-being. Awareness of how detoxification works can guide us in making dietary choices and lifestyle changes that support these processes, ultimately leading to improved health.

The Liver: The Body's Detox Workhorse

The liver is perhaps the most well-known detox organ. It performs over 500 functions daily, and many of these involve detoxification. It processes everything we eat or drink and filters out harmful substances. When you eat or drink something, your liver acts like a security guard, ensuring that any harmful agents are removed or neutralized before they can do any harm.

The liver uses two main phases for detoxification: Phase I and Phase II. In Phase I, enzymes break down toxins into smaller parts. Unfortunately, sometimes these broken-down parts can be even more harmful than the original toxin. That's where Phase II comes in—it attaches other molecules to these smaller parts to make them harmless and then sends them off to be excreted from the body.

The Kidneys: Nature's Filter

Your kidneys are another crucial part of the detox system. They constantly filter your blood, removing waste products and excess substances like water or salts. Think of your kidneys as highly efficient filtration units—they process about 120-150 quarts of blood daily to produce around 1-2 quarts of urine.

Kidneys manage this filtering process using tiny structures called nephrons. Each kidney contains around a million nephrons that filter out waste while keeping necessary elements like glucose and amino acids in your bloodstream. This filtering action helps maintain your body's fluid balance and prevents harmful waste buildup.

The Lungs: Cleansing the Breath

Our lungs serve more than just breathing in oxygen; they actively participate in expelling waste gases like carbon dioxide from our bodies. When we inhale, oxygen enters the bloodstream through tiny air sacs called alveoli. When we exhale, carbon dioxide produced by cellular metabolism leaves the body through these same air sacs.

Residents of polluted areas might face more challenges with lung detoxification due to contaminants in the air they breathe daily. However, simple practices such as deep breathing exercises or spending time in cleaner air environments can help support lung health.

The Skin: The Largest Organ's Role

Often overlooked in discussions about detoxification is the skin—the largest organ in the human body. Acting like a barrier against external toxins, it also excretes waste products through sweat. Sweating can help rid the body of heavy metals like mercury and lead.

Practices like regular exercise and saunas can boost this sweating process, helping to keep your skin healthy and functioning well as part of your overall detox system. Proper hydration is essential for this process since adequate water intake ensures that toxins are more easily swept away with sweat.

ORGAN	ROLE	METHOD
Liver	Filters blood from digestive tract	Enzyme processing (Phase I & II)
Kidneys	Filter blood to produce urine	Nephrons filtering
Lungs	Remove CO2 from blood	Exhalation
Skin	Excrete waste through sweat	Sweating

All these organs work hand-in-hand to keep our bodies free from harmful substances. By supporting their functions with a healthy diet, plenty of water, regular exercise, clean air practices, and sometimes even specific detox protocols as recommended by health professionals, we can ensure that our body's natural defense system remains robust.

CHAPTER 3

Preparing for Your Mucus Cleanse

A well-thought-out plan will set the foundation for smooth progress and sustainable results. Preparation involves not only equipping yourself with the necessary tools and knowledge but also gearing up mentally and physically.

Being mentally prepared means setting your mind on the goal, understanding why you're doing the cleanse, and visualizing the benefits you'll gain. Physical preparation includes making dietary changes, gathering any necessary supplies, and ensuring your body is ready for this transition. Every step you take beforehand will help you avoid possible pitfalls and stay committed throughout the process.

Steps to Prepare Mentally and Physically for the Cleanse

Preparing for Dr. Sebi's mucus cleanse is a journey that requires dedication and planning, both mentally and physically. To ensure success, it's essential to ready your mind and body for the changes they will undergo. Let's go through the steps in a straightforward manner.

Mental Preparation

1. **Setting Your Intention**: Identify why you want to do this cleanse. Write down your goals or even create a vision board that reminds you daily of your purpose.
2. **Educating Yourself**: Read up on Dr. Sebi's principles and the benefits of the cleanse. Understanding the reasons behind the cleanse can bolster your commitment.
3. **Visualizing Success**: Imagine yourself completing the cleanse and feeling healthier. Visualization can motivate you to adhere to the regimen when things get tough.
4. **Developing a Positive Mindset**: Replace any negative thoughts with positive affirmations. Believing in your ability to follow through is crucial.
5. **Creating a Support System**: Inform friends or family about your plans so they can offer encouragement. Joining online forums or local groups can also provide valuable support.
6. **Practical Planning**: Ensure you have time set aside each day for meal prep and relaxation exercises such as meditation or deep breathing techniques.

Physical Preparation

1. **Assessing Your Current Diet:** Take note of what you are currently eating and identify areas where you are consuming too much processed food or heavy meals.

2. **Gradual Elimination:** Remove processed foods, dairy, meat, and refined sugars from your diet gradually over a couple of weeks instead of all at once.

3. **Hydration is Key:** Increase your water intake to help flush out toxins even before starting the cleanse.

4. **Stocking Up on Essentials**: Make sure you have all necessary ingredients like fresh fruits, vegetables, herbs, and supplements recommended by Dr. Sebi.

5. **Light Exercise Routine**: Incorporate light exercise like walking or stretching into your daily routine to improve circulation and aid detoxification.

6. **Understanding Detox Symptoms:** Be aware that detox symptoms such as headaches, fatigue, or irritability may occur initially as your body adjusts.

DAILY ROUTINE ADJUSTMENT CHART		
ACTIVITY	TIME	PURPOSE
Morning Hydration	Upon Waking	Kickstart detox process
Light Exercise/Stretching	20-30 mins	Improve circulation
Meal Prep	60 mins	Ensure adherence to diet plan
Meditation/Deep Breathing	10-15 mins	Maintain mental calmness
Hydration Throughout Day	Ongoing	Continuously flush out toxins

How to Address Common Fears and Set Realistic Expectations

Maybe you're worried about whether you'll succeed, or perhaps you're unsure about what to expect. Let me reassure you—these feelings are normal. Taking on a mucus cleanse is a significant change in your lifestyle, and like any new endeavor, it comes with its set of challenges. The goal of this section is to address common fears and to help you set realistic expectations so you can approach your cleanse with confidence.

1. **Fear of Hunger and Cravings:** One of the most common fears people have is the fear of feeling hungry all the time. Many folks worry that they won't be able to satisfy their hunger on a mucus-free diet, which primarily consists of fruits, vegetables, seeds, nuts, and certain grains.

The truth is, you might feel hungry initially as your body adjusts to this new way of eating. However, consuming nutrient-dense foods will help curb those hunger pangs. Make sure you're eating enough calories from the right sources. Incorporate healthy fats like avocados and nuts into your meals to make them more filling.

2. **Fear of Social Isolation:** People often worry that following a mucus cleanse will isolate them from social situations where food plays a central role—birthday parties, family gatherings, or even simple dinner outings with friends.

The key here is preparation and communication. Let your friends and family know about your dietary changes ahead of time. You might be surprised by how supportive they can be. Moreover, many restaurants now offer plant-based options that align with a mucus-free diet. When invited to events where you think suitable food may not be available, consider bringing along something you can eat.

3. **Fear of Failure:** Many people fear they will not be able to complete the cleanse or maintain their new eating habits long-term. This fear often stems from past experiences with dieting or lifestyle changes that didn't go as planned.

It's essential to remember that this journey isn't about perfection; it's about progress. Allow yourself room for mistakes and setbacks without being too harsh on yourself. Keep your long-term health goals in mind and celebrate small victories along the way.

Realistic Expectations

1. **Initial Reactions:** Your body may react in various ways during the first few days or weeks of the cleanse. Some people experience detox symptoms like headaches, fatigue, or irritability as their bodies expel toxins.

These symptoms are usually temporary and are a sign that your body is undergoing cleansing processes. Ensure you stay hydrated by drinking plenty of water and consume soothing teas like chamomile or peppermint if needed.

2. **Weight Changes:** Another aspect many people expect immediately is weight loss. While weight loss can occur during a mucus cleanse due to reduced intake of processed foods and toxins, it's important not to focus solely on this aspect.

More critical changes are happening internally—your organs are getting healthier, inflammation is reducing, and you're likely absorbing nutrients better than before. Weight loss may come naturally as a secondary benefit over time.

3. **Energy Levels:** You might find your energy levels fluctuating during the initial phases of the cleanse. This fluctuation happens because your body is adapting itself to derive energy from different sources—primarily fruits and vegetables instead of processed foods laden with sugar and unhealthy fats.

Over time, many people find that they have higher energy levels than before starting the cleanse since whole foods provide sustained energy throughout the day without crashes.

4. **Visualizing Success**: Creating a daily routine can also help alleviate some fears while setting expectations:

   a) *Morning Routine:* Start your day with warm lemon water. This habit helps kickstart your metabolism and flush out toxins. Follow it up with a fruit-based breakfast, such as a smoothie or a bowl of mixed fruits.
   b) *Mid-Morning Snack:* Opt for a handful of nuts or seeds. These are great sources of healthy fats and protein, helping you stay satiated until lunch.
   c) *Lunch:* A big salad filled with diverse vegetables is an excellent lunchtime choice. Adding avocados provides healthy fats that keep you feeling full.
   d) *Afternoon Routine:* A blended smoothie or freshly squeezed juice can give you an energy boost during the afternoon slump. Keep it balanced with greens, fruits, and perhaps some chia seeds.
   e) *Dinner:* For dinner, consider having vegetable soup or a vegetable stir-fry paired with quinoa or brown rice. These meals are not only nutritious but also comforting and filling.
   f) *Evening Routine:* Unwind in the evening with some calming herbal tea like chamomile or peppermint. If you're feeling peckish before bed, a light fruit snack should suffice.

TIME	ACTIVITY
Morning	Lemon water followed by fruit-based breakfast
Mid-Morning	Light snack (nuts or seeds)
Lunch	Large salad with a variety of vegetables and avocado

Afternoon	Smoothie or fresh juice
Dinner	Vegetable soup or stir-fry with quinoa or brown rice
Evening	Herbal tea and light fruit snack

Remember to drink plenty of water throughout the day to stay hydrated and support your body's detoxification processes. Building these habits gradually diminishes fears, sets the stage for realistic expectations, and ultimately leads to a more successful cleanse experience.

Guidelines for Transitioning to a Plant-Based Diet

It's not just about changing what you eat but also about shifting how you approach nutrition and wellness in your daily life. I've assembled these guidelines to smooth your transition, ensuring that you're well-prepared to embrace this lifestyle change and reap its extensive benefits.

It's essential to understand why you're making the switch. Whether it's for health reasons, environmental concerns, or ethical motivations, keeping your reason in mind will help you stay focused and committed.

1. **Start Gradually:** Transitioning doesn't have to happen overnight. Begin by incorporating more plant-based foods into your existing diet. For instance, replace milk with almond or oat milk, add more vegetables to your meals, and explore plant-based snacks like nuts and fruits.

2. **Education and Planning**: Knowledge is power. Educate yourself about the nutritional aspects of a plant-based diet. Understand where you'll get vital nutrients like protein, iron, calcium, and vitamin B12. Planning meals ahead of time can help ensure that you're not missing out on these essential nutrients.

3. **Stock Your Pantry**: A well-stocked pantry is crucial for success. Fill it with whole grains like quinoa and brown rice, legumes such as beans and lentils, nuts, seeds, and an array of spices. These staples form the backbone of a plant-based diet.

4. **Meal Prep**: Cooking at home rather than dining out allows you complete control over what goes into your food. Set aside time each week to prepare meals in bulk. Batch cooking can make weekday meals quick and easy, reducing the temptation to reach for less healthy options.

5. **Listen to Your Body:** Pay attention to how your body feels during the transition. Some people might experience slight digestive changes as their bodies adjust to increased fiber

intake from fruits, vegetables, whole grains, and legumes. This is normal; stay hydrated and give your body time to adapt.

6. **Find Plant-Based Protein Sources**: Protein is vital for building and repairing tissues. Good plant-based protein sources include lentils, chickpeas, black beans, tofu, tempeh, edamame, quinoa, chia seeds, hemp seeds, almonds, and walnuts.

7. **Balanced Meals**: Ensure that each meal is well-balanced with a diversity of nutrients:

NUTRIENT	PLANT-BASED SOURCES
Protein	Lentils, chickpeas, tofu
Iron	Spinach, lentils
Calcium	Almonds, sesame seeds
Vitamin B12	Fortified cereals
Omega-3 Fatty Acids	Flaxseeds

8. **Transition at Your Own Pace**: Everyone's journey is different. Some might find it easy to go fully plant-based quickly while others may need more time. Find what works best for you without pressuring yourself to make drastic changes all at once.

9. **Seek Support**: Join plant-based communities either online or in person where you can share experiences & recipes and get support. Having a network can be incredibly motivating.

10. **Experiment with Recipes**: Variety keeps things interesting! Try new recipes regularly. The internet offers a plethora of resources—blogs, videos & cookbooks specifically tailored to plant-based eating can be invaluable tools.

11. **Be Mindful When Eating Out**: Research restaurants ahead of time for their plant-based options or seek places known for offering vegan/vegetarian menus. Don't hesitate to ask servers if certain dishes can be modified to fit your new dietary needs.

12. **Supplementation if Needed**: Depending on individual needs or food availability in certain regions; supplementation might be needed especially for Vitamin B12 & Omega-3 fatty acids (DHA/EPA). Consult with health professionals to find out what supplements, if any, you should take to ensure that your nutritional needs are being fully met.

It's okay to make mistakes along the way. Transitioning to a plant-based diet is a learning process, and it's normal to experience ups and downs. Remind yourself of the benefits that led you to make this change and keep moving forward, even if you sometimes take small steps back.

Here's a simple guide to get started with some plant-based food swaps:

SWAP THIS	FOR THIS
Cow's Milk	Almond Milk, Oat Milk
Beef Burgers	Black Bean Burgers
Chicken	Tofu or Tempeh
Cheese	Nutritional Yeast
Butter	Coconut Oil or Avocado

Read books, watch documentaries, and follow social media influencers who advocate for plant-based living. Keeping yourself inspired will make the transition more enjoyable and less like a chore. Regular check-ups with your doctor can ensure that you're meeting your nutritional needs and maintaining overall health. Blood tests can help monitor crucial nutrients like iron and B12.

Remember, transitioning to a plant-based diet is not just about food; it's about creating a healthier lifestyle for yourself. Take it one step at a time and celebrate your progress along the way. Stay committed, stay informed, and most importantly, enjoy the journey towards better health!

Get Your __Free__ Bonuses Now

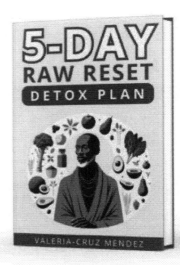 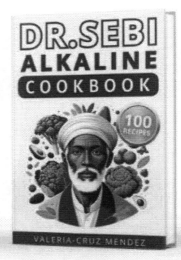 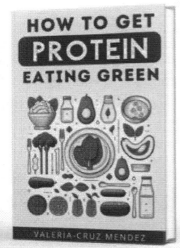

BONUS #1: 5-Day Raw Reset Detox Plan

Jumpstart your journey to wellness with **a 5-day detox plan** designed to cleanse your body, reset your system, and boost your energy levels, all while staying true to Dr. Sebi's principles.

BONUS #2: Dr. Sebi Alkaline Cookbook

Delve into over **100 mouth-watering alkaline recipes** that not only adhere to the alkaline diet but also turn every meal into a healing, nutritious feast for your body.

BONUS #3: How to Get Protein Eating Green

Discover the secrets of **meeting your protein needs with plant-based sources**, ensuring your nutrition is holistic, sustainable, and perfectly aligned with an alkaline lifestyle.

Scan with your phone's camera **OR** go to:

https://shorturl.at/gjpy8

CHAPTER 4

28-Day Dr. Sebi Mucus Cleanse Detox Plan

The Dr. Sebi Mucus Cleanse Detox Plan is a cleansing regimen designed to rid the body of excess mucus and toxins. Based on the teachings of Dr. Sebi, a renowned herbalist and healer, this plan emphasizes the use of natural foods and herbs to purify the body and enhance overall well-being.

It is believed that excess mucus in the body can lead to various health issues, including respiratory problems, inflammation, and compromised immune function. By eliminating this mucus, the body can function more efficiently, leading to improved health, increased energy levels, and a greater sense of vitality.

This cleanse is not just about what you eat but also involves mental and emotional preparation. It's important to stay motivated and focused on your goals for the best results.

Week 1: Transition Phase

. This week is the Transition Phase, where we slowly start to shift our habits and prepare our bodies for the deeper cleansing that will follow. The goal is to gradually reduce the intake of processed foods, sugars, and other toxins to ease your body into the coming changes.

Day 1-3: Initial Adjustments

The first three days are all about making small but significant changes. Start by drinking a glass of water with lemon every morning. This simple habit helps kickstart your digestive system and begins to flush out toxins.

Day 4-7: Clean Eating Basics

As you move further into the week, start replacing one meal a day with a plant-based option. Whether it's a salad for lunch or a vegetable soup for dinner, focus on incorporating whole foods that are as close to their natural state as possible. Avoid caffeine, alcohol, and sugary drinks. Opt for herbal teas or water instead.

SAMPLE SCHEDULE FOR WEEK 1			
DAY	**MORNING**	**MIDDAY**	**EVENING**
1-3	Warm lemon water	Plant-based snack (fruit/nuts)	Vegetable broth or light salad
4-7	Smoothie with greens	Whole grain bowl with vegetables	Steamed veggies or plant-based protein

Week 2: Deep Cleansing

In Week 2, we dive deeper into the cleansing process. This is where the real detoxification happens, so it's important to stay committed and listen to your body's needs.

Day 8-10: Juicing & Smoothies

Begin incorporating more liquids into your diet through juices and smoothies. These are nutrient-dense and help in flushing out toxins efficiently. A green juice in the morning and a fruit smoothie in the afternoon can work wonders.

Day 11-14: Raw Foods Only

To maximize detoxification, switch to an all-raw diet for these four days. Fresh fruits, vegetables, nuts, and seeds should make up your meals. This can be challenging but think of it as giving your digestive system a much-needed break.

SAMPLE SCHEDULE FOR WEEK 2			
DAY	**MORNING**	**MIDDAY**	**EVENING**
8-10	Green juice	Fruit smoothie	Light raw salad
11-14	Fresh fruit platter	Mixed green salad	Raw veggie stir-fry

Week 3: Fasting & Reset

This is perhaps the most intense part of our cleanse—the fasting period. Fasting helps reset your system and promotes autophagy, where cells clean out damaged components and regenerate new ones.

Day 15-18: Intermittent Fasting

Start with intermittent fasting. Limit eating to an eight-hour window during the day and fast for the remaining sixteen hours. Drink plenty of water, herbal teas, and light broths during fasting periods.

Day 19-21: Full Fasting (Optional)

If you feel ready, transition into full fasting by consuming only liquids—water, herbal teas, vegetable broths—throughout these days. Monitor how you feel closely; if you experience any severe discomforts, ease back to intermittent fasting.

SAMPLE SCHEDULE FOR WEEK 3		
DAY	EATING WINDOW	FASTING HOURS
5-18	Noon 8 PM	All other hours
19-21	Liquids only	All hours (if opted)

Week 4: Reintroduction & Maintenance

As we enter the final week of our 28-day cleanse, reintroducing certain foods is key to maintaining the benefits we've achieved. The objective this week is to gradually integrate solid foods while still focusing on clean, nutritious options.

Day 22-24: Gradual Reintroduction

Start by adding easily digestible foods back into your diet. Think steamed vegetables, brown rice, and quinoa. This slow reintroduction helps your digestive system adjust without overwhelming it.

Day 25-28: Balanced Meals

Continue to incorporate more variety into your meals while maintaining a balanced diet rich in fruits, vegetables, whole grains, and lean proteins. Avoid processed foods, refined sugars, and excessive caffeine.

SAMPLE SCHEDULE FOR WEEK 4			
DAY	MORNING	MIDDAY	EVENING

22-24	Smoothie with fruits and nuts	Steamed vegetables with brown rice	Quinoa bowl with veggies
25-28	Fresh fruit smoothie	Mixed grain salad	Baked sweet potato with greens

Congratulations on completing this transformative 28-day cleanse! Remember, the key to lasting benefits is adopting these healthy habits into your everyday life. Stay mindful of your food choices and listen to your body as you continue this wellness journey.

Incorporation of Specific Dr. Sebi-approved Herbs and Foods

Below are the specific herbs and foods approved by Dr. Sebi and how you can incorporate them into your diet. These changes are not just about food; they signify a step towards purifying your body for optimal health.

Morning Routine

1. **Burdock Root:** Start your day with a burdock root tea. Known for its blood-purifying properties, burdock root helps get rid of toxins from the bloodstream.
2. **Dandelion Root**: Dandelion root tea can be another great addition to your morning routine. It aids in liver detoxification and supports digestion.
3. **Fruits:** Begin with consuming fresh fruits like berries, oranges, or apples which are alkaline and rich in fiber.
4. **Smoothie:** Create a green smoothie using ingredients such as kale, spinach, avocado, hemp seeds, and Dr. Sebi-approved fruits like banana or strawberry.

Mid-Morning Snack

1. **Nuts:** Snack on raw almonds or walnuts which provide good fats and essential nutrients.
2. **Sea Moss Gel:** Sea moss is packed with vitamins and minerals; adding a spoonful of sea moss gel to your snack can boost your nutrient intake.

Lunch

1. **Nettle Leaves:** Nettle leaf tea at lunch helps reduce inflammation and build strong bones.
2. **Anise Seed:** Adding anise seeds to your meals can enhance digestion.
3. **Green Salad:** Prepare a large salad with mixed greens like arugula, lettuce, cucumbers, bell peppers, onions topped with sesame seeds.

4. **Quinoa/Brown Rice:** Pair your salad with whole grains like quinoa or brown rice for added protein.

Afternoon Snack

1. **Fruit Bowl:** A small bowl of seasonal fruits like mangoes or grapes.
2. **Veggie Sticks with Hummus:** Carrot and celery sticks dipped in organic hummus make for a crunchy treat.

Dinner

1. **Sarsaparilla:** Consuming a tea made from sarsaparilla root can help purify the blood and improve skin health.
2. **Ginger Root:** Incorporate ginger root in your meals to boost digestion.
3. **Veggie Stir-fry:** Sauté vegetables such as zucchini, broccoli, bell peppers in olive oil with lots of garlic and ginger.
4. **Chickpeas/Lentils:** Complement the stir-fry with legumes like chickpeas or lentils that provide protein without being acidic.

Evening Wind Down

1. **Chamomile Tea:** End the day with chamomile tea to help relax and promote good sleep.

Integrating these herbs and foods really heightens my sense of balance during the cleanse period by continuously promoting the elimination of unwanted mucus from the body.

Tips for Managing Detox Symptoms and Staying Motivated

It's normal to experience some detox symptoms as your body adjusts to the new lifestyle and begins to cleanse itself. Detoxing can sometimes be uncomfortable, but understanding what's happening in your body can help you stay positive. When you begin a detox, your body starts to release stored toxins. This can cause fatigue, headaches, irritability, and other symptoms. Knowing that these are signs that your body is healing can make them more manageable.

Managing Detox Symptoms

1. **Hydrate Often:** Drinking plenty of water is essential during a detox. Water helps flush out toxins more effectively and keeps you hydrated. Avoid sugary drinks and stick to water or herbal teas. I try to drink at least 8-10 glasses of water daily to keep things moving smoothly.

2. **Rest is Essential:** Your body works hard during detoxification, and getting enough rest is important. Make sleep a priority—aim for at least 7-8 hours per night. If you feel tired during the day, don't hesitate to take short naps.

3. **Eat Healing Foods:** Eating foods rich in nutrients helps support your body's detox processes. Focus on consuming a variety of fruits and vegetables. Alkaline foods recommended by Dr. Sebi can be particularly beneficial for their cleansing properties.

4. **Exercise Moderately:** Light physical activity like walking or yoga can help stimulate lymphatic flow and aid in the elimination of toxins. Be careful not to overdo it; listen to your body and rest when needed.

5. **Warm Baths:** Taking warm baths with Epsom salt can ease muscle aches and promote relaxation. Adding essential oils like lavender or eucalyptus can enhance the soothing effect.

Staying Motivated

Detoxing isn't always easy but staying motivated is key to reaping the benefits in the long run. Here are some tips that have helped me maintain focus:

1. **Set Clear Goals:** Remember why you started this journey in the first place. Write down your goals and refer back to them when you're feeling discouraged.

2. **Track Your Progress:** Keeping a journal or using an app to track your progress can be encouraging as you see changes over time—be it improved energy levels, clearer skin, or better digestion.

3. **Join a Support Group:** Connecting with others who are also following Dr. Sebi's Mucus Cleanse can provide much-needed support and motivation. Sharing experiences and tips with like-minded individuals makes the journey less lonely.

4. **Stay Informed:** Educate yourself continuously about the benefits of detoxing and alkaline foods by reading books or articles on the subject., Knowledge empowers you to make better choices and reinforces why you're doing this cleanse.

CHAPTER 5

Recipes & Meal Plans

Breakfast Recipes

Quinoa Porridge with Fresh Berries

Preparation time: 10 mins

Cooking time: 20 mins

Servings: 2

Ingredients:

- One cup quinoa
- Two cups water
- One cup fresh mixed berries (blueberries, strawberries, raspberries)
- Two tbsp agave syrup
- One tsp vanilla extract
- One tbsp chia seeds

Directions:

1. Rinse the quinoa under cold water. In a medium saucepan, bring the two cups of water to a boil.

2. Add the quinoa to the boiling water, then adjust to low temp. Cover and simmer for about 15 mins or until the water is absorbed and the quinoa is tender.

3. Remove, then stir in the vanilla extract and agave syrup. Divide the quinoa porridge into bowls and top with fresh mixed berries. Sprinkle each serving with chia seeds.

Tips: You can soak the quinoa overnight for easier digestion. Feel free to switch up the berries as per the season.

Serving size: One bowl

Nutritional values (per serving): Calories: 300; Fat: 6g; Carbs: 58g; Protein: 8g; Sodium: 10mg; Sugar: 12g; Cholesterol: 0mg; Fiber: 7g

Apple-Cinnamon Quinoa Breakfast Bake

Preparation time: 10 mins

Cooking time: 30 mins

Servings: 4

Ingredients:

- One cup quinoa
- Two cups water
- One apple, chopped
- Two tsp cinnamon
- One tbsp agave syrup
- Half cup walnuts, chopped

- Pinch of sea salt

Directions:

1. Warm up your oven to 375°F. Rinse and drain quinoa. In a pot, let quinoa and water boil, reduce heat, then simmer for 15 mins.
2. In a bowl, mix cooked quinoa, chopped apple, cinnamon, agave syrup, walnuts, and sea salt. Transfer mixture to a baking dish.
3. Bake for 15 mins, then let it cool before serving.

Tips: You can add some berries for extra flavor before baking.

Serving size: One cup

Nutritional values (per serving): Calories: 250; Fat: 8g; Carbs: 38g; Protein: 6g; Sodium: 50mg; Sugar: 10g; Cholesterol: 0mg; Fiber: 5g

Soursop Smoothie with Chia Seeds

Preparation time: 10 mins

Cooking time: N/A

Servings: 2

Ingredients:

- One cup soursop pulp
- Two tbsp chia seeds
- One cup coconut milk
- One banana
- One tbsp agave nectar

Directions:

1. Scoop the soursop pulp into a blender. Add the chia seeds, coconut milk, banana, and agave nectar to the blender.
2. Blend on high until smooth and creamy. Pour into glasses and serve immediately.

Tips: You can refrigerate the soursop pulp for about half an hour before blending for a colder smoothie. Add ice cubes to make it more refreshing.

Serving size: 1 glass

Nutritional values (per serving): Calories: 220; Fat: 9g; Carbs: 35g; Protein: 3g; Sodium: 60mg; Sugar: 22g; Cholesterol: 0mg; Fiber: 7g

Dr. Sebi's Banana Walnut Bread

Preparation time: 15 mins

Cooking time: 60 mins

Servings: 8 slices

Ingredients:

- Two cups spelt flour
- Three bananas, mashed
- Half cup walnuts, chopped
- Quarter cup agave nectar

- Quarter cup coconut oil, melted
- One tsp baking powder
- One tsp sea salt

Directions:

1. Warm up your oven to 350°F. Grease a loaf pan with a little coconut oil.
2. In your big container, mix spelt flour, baking powder, and sea salt. Mash the bananas in a separate bowl and then add the agave nectar and melted coconut oil.
3. Mix the wet ingredients into the dry ingredients until just combined. Fold in the chopped walnuts gently. Pour the batter into the greased loaf pan, spreading it evenly.
4. Bake for about one hour or until a toothpick inserted into the center comes out clean. Allow to cool in the pan for about ten mins before transferring to a wire rack to cool completely.

Tips: For extra crunch, sprinkle some chopped walnuts on top before baking. Make sure not to overmix the batter to keep the bread light and fluffy.

Serving size: 1 slice

Nutritional values (per serving): Calories: 180; Fat: 9g; Carbs: 23g; Protein: 4g; Sodium: 150mg; Sugar: 8g; Cholesterol: 0mg; Fiber: 3g

Chia Seed Pudding with Agave Syrup

Preparation time: 15 mins + overnight chilling

Cooking time: N/A

Servings: 2

Ingredients:

- Four tbsp chia seeds
- Two cups almond milk (or other plant-based milk)
- Two tbsp agave syrup
- One tsp vanilla extract
- Fresh fruit for topping (optional)

Directions:

1. In your medium container, mix almond milk, chia seeds, agave syrup, and vanilla extract. Stir well until thoroughly combined.
2. Let it sit for about 10 mins, then stir again to prevent clumping. Cover the bowl and refrigerate overnight or for at least four hours.
3. Before serving, stir the pudding again to ensure even consistency. Divide into serving bowls and top with fresh fruit if desired.

Tips: For a creamier texture, you can blend the mixture before chilling. Add a pinch of sea moss gel for added nutritional benefits.

Serving size: One cup

Nutritional values (per serving): Calories: 250; Fat: 12g; Carbs: 30g; Protein: 7g; Sodium: 60mg; Sugar: 12g; Cholesterol: 0mg; Fiber: 14g

Alkaline Green Power Juice

Preparation time: 10 mins

Cooking time: N/A

Servings: 2

Ingredients:

- One cup kale
- One cup cucumber
- One cup green apple, chopped
- Two tbsp fresh lemon juice
- One tsp fresh ginger, grated
- One cup spring water
- One tbsp agave syrup (optional)

Directions:

1. Thoroughly wash all the ingredients. Mix kale, cucumber, green apple, lemon juice, ginger, and spring water in a blender. Blend until smooth.
2. If desired, add agave syrup to sweeten and blend for an additional 15 seconds. Strain the mixture through a fine mesh strainer to remove pulp for a smoother texture.

Tips: Drink immediately after preparation to maximize nutrient intake. You can use ice-cold spring water for a refreshing twist.

Serving size: One cup

Nutritional values (per serving): Calories: 60; Fat: 0g; Carbs: 15g; Protein: 1g; Sodium: 10mg; Sugar: 10g; Cholesterol: 0mg; Fiber: 2g

Butternut Squash Hash Browns

Preparation time: 15 mins

Cooking time: 20 mins

Servings: 4

Ingredients:

- One butternut squash, peeled and grated (approx. three cups)
- Two tbsp avocado oil
- One tsp sea salt
- One tsp onion powder
- Half tsp garlic powder
- One tsp dried thyme
- One tbsp chopped fresh parsley

Directions:

1. Peel and grate the butternut squash. In a large bowl, mix the grated squash with sea salt, onion powder, garlic powder, and dried thyme.
2. Heat the avocado oil in a large skillet on moderate temp. Add the squash mixture to the skillet, spreading it out evenly.
3. Cook for about ten mins on one side or until golden brown. Flip and cook the other side for an additional ten

mins or until thoroughly cooked. Remove, then garnish with fresh parsley.

Tips: Be sure to squeeze out excess moisture from the grated squash to ensure crispy hash browns.

Serving size: 1 cup

Nutritional values (per serving): Calories: 120; Fat: 10g; Carbs: 12g; Protein: 1g; Sodium: 400mg; Sugar: 3g; Cholesterol: 0mg; Fiber: 3g

Teff Pancakes with Agave Syrup

Preparation time: 10 mins

Cooking time: 20 mins

Servings: 4

Ingredients:

- One cup teff flour
- One tsp baking powder
- One tbsp agave syrup
- One cup spring water
- Two tbsp coconut oil (for cooking)
- A pinch of sea salt

Directions:

1. In a large bowl, mix the teff flour, baking powder, and sea salt. Gradually add in the spring water while stirring to create a smooth batter.

2. Heat the coconut oil in a skillet on moderate temp. Pour about one-fourth cup of batter into the skillet for each pancake.

3. Cook until bubbles appear on the surface, then flip and cook until both sides are golden brown. Drizzle agave syrup over the pancakes before serving.

Tips: For extra flavor, add a pinch of cinnamon to the batter.

Serving size: Two pancakes

Nutritional values (per serving): Calories: 180; Fat: 5g; Carbs: 30g; Protein: 3g; Sodium: 90mg; Sugar: 6g; Cholesterol: 0mg; Fiber: 2g

Spelt Flour Banana Muffins

Preparation time: 15 mins

Cooking time: 25 mins

Servings: 12 muffins

Ingredients:

- Two cups spelt flour
- Three ripe bananas, mashed
- One tsp baking soda
- One tbsp agave syrup
- Half cup coconut milk
- Two tbsp grapeseed oil
- A pinch of sea salt

Directions:

1. Preheat your oven to 350°F and line a muffin tin with paper liners. In a medium bowl, mix the spelt flour, baking soda, and sea salt.

2. In another bowl, combine the mashed bananas, agave syrup, coconut milk, and grapeseed oil. Gradually fold the wet ingredients into the dry ingredients until just combined.

3. Spoon the batter evenly into the muffin cups. Bake for twenty-five mins or until a toothpick inserted into the center comes out clean. Let cool before serving.

Tips: Add chopped nuts or dried fruit for added texture.

Serving size: One muffin

Nutritional values (per serving): Calories: 130; Fat: 4g; Carbs: 22g; Protein: 2g; Sodium: 95mg; Sugar: 5g; Cholesterol: 0mg; Fiber: 3g

Sea Moss and Bladderwrack Smoothie

Preparation time: 10 mins

Cooking time: N/A

Servings: 2

Ingredients:

- Two tbsp dried sea moss gel
- One tbsp bladderwrack powder
- One banana
- One cup blueberries
- Two cups coconut milk
- One tbsp agave syrup

Directions:

1. Add the banana, blueberries, coconut milk, sea moss gel, and bladderwrack powder into a blender. Blend until smooth and creamy.

2. If desired, add the agave syrup for extra sweetness and blend briefly to mix.

Tips: For best results, prepare the sea moss gel ahead by soaking dried sea moss in water overnight and then blending it with fresh water until smooth. This smoothie is perfect as a morning energizer or post-workout refreshment.

Serving size: One cup

Nutritional values (per serving): Calories: 120; Fat: 4g; Carbs: 22g; Protein: 2g; Sodium: 5mg; Sugar: 12g; Cholesterol: 0mg; Fiber: 3g

Lunch Recipes

Bell Pepper and Avocado Wraps

Preparation time: 10 mins

Cooking time: N/A

Servings: 4

Ingredients:

- Two large bell peppers (any color), thinly sliced (approx. two cups)
- Two ripe avocados, pitted and sliced
- Four large collard green leaves
- One tbsp lime juice
- Half tsp sea salt
- Half tsp black pepper
- One tbsp extra virgin olive oil

Directions:

1. Wash and pat dry the collard green leaves. Thinly slice the bell peppers and avocados.
2. In a bowl, combine the bell pepper slices, lime juice, olive oil, sea salt, and black pepper. Lay each collard green leaf flat and add an equal amount of sliced avocado.
3. Top with the bell pepper mixture. Roll up each leaf like a wrap.

Tips: You can secure the wraps with toothpicks to keep them from unrolling.

Serving size: 1 wrap

Nutritional values (per serving): Calories: 180; Fat: 14g; Carbs: 12g; Protein: 2g; Sodium: 350mg; Sugar: 3g; Cholesterol: 0mg; Fiber: 7g

Cauliflower Rice with Tempeh Stir-fry

Preparation time: 15 mins

Cooking time: 20 mins

Servings: 4

Ingredients:

- One lb. cauliflower
- One lb. tempeh
- Two tbsp coconut oil
- Two cloves garlic, minced
- One bell pepper, chopped
- Two tbsp tamari (or other soy sauce alternative)
- One tsp sea salt

Directions:

1. Break the cauliflower into florets and pulse in a food processor until it resembles rice. Cut the tempeh into bite-sized pieces.
2. Heat coconut oil in a large skillet on moderate temp. Add garlic, then sauté until fragrant. Add the tempeh pieces and cook for five mins, until browned on all sides.
3. Add the chopped bell pepper and continue to cook for another five mins. Stir in the cauliflower rice and tamari, mixing well.
4. Season with sea salt and cook for another five mins, stirring occasionally.

Tips: You can add other vegetables like zucchini or carrots for more variety. Serve with a sprinkle of sesame seeds for added texture.

Serving size: 1 cup

Nutritional values (per serving): Calories: 180; Fat: 11g; Carbs: 12g; Protein: 10g; Sodium: 400mg; Sugar: 2g; Cholesterol: 0mg; Fiber: 4g

Roasted Garlic and Tomato Soup

Preparation time: 10 mins

Cooking time: 40 mins

Servings: 4

Ingredients:

- Two lbs. tomatoes, halved
- One bulb garlic, top sliced off
- Two tbsp olive oil
- One tsp sea salt
- One tsp black pepper
- Four cups vegetable broth
- One tbsp fresh basil, chopped

Directions:

1. Warm up your oven to 400°F. Place the halved tomatoes and garlic bulb on a baking sheet. Drizzle with olive oil, sea salt, and black pepper.
2. Roast in the oven for thirty mins, until tomatoes are soft and garlic is aromatic. Remove, then cool slightly.

3. In a blender, combine roasted tomatoes, squeezed out roasted garlic cloves, and vegetable broth. Blend until smooth, then transfer to a large pot.
4. Heat on moderate temp and bring to a simmer for about ten mins. Stir in fresh basil before serving.

Tips: For an extra creamy texture, you can blend in half an avocado before heating.

Serving size: 1 cup

Nutritional values (per serving): Calories: 110; Fat: 7g; Carbs: 11g; Protein: 2g; Sodium: 600mg; Sugar: 6g; Cholesterol: 0mg; Fiber: 3g

Wild Rice and Bell Pepper Stir-Fry

Preparation time: 10 mins

Cooking time: 30 mins

Servings: 4

Ingredients:

- Two cups wild rice, cooked
- One red bell pepper, sliced
- One green bell pepper, sliced
- One yellow bell pepper, sliced
- Two tbsp olive oil
- Two cloves garlic, minced
- One tsp sea salt

Directions:

1. Heat the olive oil in a large skillet over medium-high heat. Add the minced garlic and sauté for one minute until fragrant.
2. Add the bell peppers and cook for five to seven mins until tender. Stir in the cooked wild rice and sea salt.
3. Cook for an additional three to five mins, stirring frequently. Adjust seasoning as necessary before serving.

Tips: Use fresh, organic vegetables for the best results. You can substitute bell peppers with other Dr. Sebi-approved vegetables if desired.

Serving size: One cup

Nutritional values (per serving): Calories: 200; Fat: 7g; Carbs: 33g; Protein: 6g; Sodium: 350mg; Sugar: 5g; Cholesterol: 0mg; Fiber: 6g

Butternut Squash Soup with Ginger

Preparation time: 15 mins

Cooking time: 25 mins

Servings: 4

Ingredients:

- Two cups butternut squash, cubed
- One tbsp fresh ginger, grated
- Four cups vegetable broth (Dr. Sebi-approved)
- One onion, chopped
- Two tbsp olive oil
- One tsp sea salt

Directions:

1. Heat olive oil in a large pot on moderate temp. Add chopped onion and cook for five mins until translucent.
2. Add butternut squash cubes and grated ginger, then sauté for two to three mins. Pour in broth, then let it boil.
3. Reduce the heat and let it simmer for fifteen to twenty mins until squash is tender. Use an immersion blender to puree the soup until smooth. Flavor it with sea salt.

Tips: Garnish with fresh herbs such as cilantro or parsley for added flavor.

Serving size: One cup

Nutritional values (per serving): Calories: 150; Fat: 8g; Carbs: 22g; Protein: 3g; Sodium: 600mg; Sugar: 5g; Cholesterol: 0mg; Fiber: 4g

Portobello Mushroom Burgers

Preparation time: Fifteen mins

Cooking time: Fifteen mins

Servings: Four

Ingredients:

- Four large portobello mushrooms

- Two tbsp olive oil
- One tsp sea salt
- One tsp black pepper
- Half cup arugula
- One avocado, sliced
- Four whole-grain burger buns

Directions:

1. Warm up your grill to medium-high heat. Remove stems from portobello mushrooms and brush both sides with olive oil.
2. Flavor mushrooms with sea salt and black pepper. Place mushrooms on the grill, gill side down, and cook for five to seven mins per side until tender.
3. Toast the whole-grain burger buns on the grill for two mins. Assemble the burgers by placing one grilled mushroom on each bun, followed by arugula and avocado slices.

Tips: Add a squeeze of lemon juice on the avocado for extra flavor. Serve immediately to enjoy the best texture.

Serving size: One burger

Nutritional values (per serving): Calories: 240; Fat: 14g; Carbs: 22g; Protein: 5g; Sodium: 390mg; Sugar: 3g; Cholesterol: 0mg; Fiber: 6g

Spicy Lentil Soup with Cayenne Pepper

Preparation time: Ten mins

Cooking time: Thirty-five mins

Servings: Four

Ingredients:

- One cup red lentils, rinsed
- Six cups vegetable broth
- One tbsp olive oil
- One large onion, chopped
- Two cloves garlic, minced
- One tsp cayenne pepper
- One tsp sea salt

Directions:

1. In a large pot, heat olive oil on moderate temp. Add chopped onion and cook for five mins until translucent.
2. Stir in minced garlic and cook for an additional minute. Add red lentils, vegetable broth, cayenne pepper, and sea salt to the pot.
3. Let it boil, then simmer for thirty mins until lentils are tender. Use an immersion blender to blend soup to desired consistency or leave it chunky as preferred.

Tips: Garnish with fresh cilantro or parsley for added freshness. Adjust the cayenne pepper quantity based on your spice preference.

Serving size: One cup

Nutritional values (per serving): Calories: 180; Fat: 4g; Carbs: 28g; Protein: 9g; Sodium: 700mg; Sugar: 3g; Cholesterol: 0mg; Fiber: 8g

Grilled Portobello Mushrooms with Herbs

Preparation time: Twenty mins

Cooking time: Fifteen mins

Servings: Four

Ingredients:

- Four large Portobello mushrooms
- Two tbsp olive oil
- One tbsp lemon juice
- One tsp sea salt
- One tsp black pepper
- Two cloves garlic, minced
- One tbsp fresh thyme leaves

Directions:

1. Preheat the grill to medium-high heat. In a small bowl, mix olive oil, lemon juice, sea salt, black pepper, and minced garlic.
2. Brush both sides of the mushroom caps with the mixture. Place mushrooms on the grill and cook for about seven mins on each side or until tender.

3. Sprinkle fresh thyme leaves over the mushrooms before serving.

Tips: For added flavor, you can marinate the mushrooms in the mixture for up to one hour before grilling.

Serving size: One mushroom cap

Nutritional values (per serving): Calories: 88; Fat: 7g; Carbs: 5g; Protein: 3g; Sodium: 200mg; Sugar: 2g; Cholesterol: 0mg; Fiber: 2g

Raw Kale and Avocado Salad

Preparation time: Fifteen mins

Cooking time: N/A

Servings: Four

Ingredients:

- Four cups chopped kale leaves (stems removed)
- One large avocado, diced
- Juice of one lemon
- One tbsp olive oil
- Half tsp sea salt
- Quarter tsp black pepper
- Two tbsp pumpkin seeds

Directions:

1. In a large bowl, add chopped kale and drizzle with lemon juice and olive oil. Using your hands, massage the kale for about two mins until it softens.

2. Add diced avocado and mix gently to combine. Sprinkle sea salt, black pepper, and pumpkin seeds over the salad. Toss gently to mix well before serving.

Tips: For an extra crunch, you can add more seeds or nuts of your choice.

Serving size: One cup

Nutritional values (per serving): Calories: 154; Fat: 11g; Carbs: 13g; Protein: 3g; Sodium: 200mg; Sugar: 1g; Cholesterol: 0mg; Fiber: 6g

Sautéed Zucchini and Squash Medley

Preparation time: 10 mins

Cooking time: 15 mins

Servings: 4

Ingredients:

- Two zucchinis, sliced
- Two yellow squashes, sliced
- Two tbsp olive oil
- Four cloves garlic, minced
- One tsp sea salt
- One tsp black pepper
- One tbsp fresh parsley, chopped

Directions:

1. Heat olive oil in a large skillet on moderate temp. Add garlic to the skillet and sauté until fragrant. Add

sliced zucchinis and yellow squashes to the pan.

2. Flavor it with sea salt and black pepper. Cook until vegetables are tender but still crisp. Sprinkle with fresh parsley before serving.

Tips: Avoid overcooking to maintain the crisp texture of the vegetables. Pair this dish with a light salad for a complete meal.

Serving size: One cup

Nutritional values (per serving): Calories: 100; Fat: 7g; Carbs: 8g; Protein: 2g; Sodium: 180mg; Sugar: 4g; Cholesterol: 0mg; Fiber: 2g

Dinner Recipes

Zucchini Noodles with Tahini Sauce

Preparation time: 15 mins

Cooking time: N/A

Servings: 2

Ingredients:

- Two medium zucchinis
- One-fourth cup tahini
- Two tbsp lemon juice
- One tbsp maple syrup
- One clove garlic, minced
- One-fourth cup water

- Salt to taste

Directions:

1. Spiralize the zucchinis to create zucchini noodles.
2. In a bowl, whisk together the tahini, lemon juice, maple syrup, minced garlic, water, and salt until smooth.
3. Toss the zucchini noodles with the tahini sauce until evenly coated. Serve immediately or chill in the refrigerator for 10 mins before serving.

Tips: Add a sprinkle of sesame seeds on top for extra crunch. For added flavor, include fresh herbs like parsley or cilantro.

Serving size: One cup

Nutritional values (per serving): Calories: 180; Fat: 12g; Carbs: 15g; Protein: 5g; Sodium: 150mg; Sugar: 6g; Cholesterol: 0mg; Fiber: 4g

Chickpea and Spinach Stew

Preparation time: 10 mins

Cooking time: 20 mins

Servings: 4

Ingredients:

- One lb. cooked chickpeas (about two cups)
- Six cups fresh spinach
- Two cups vegetable broth

- One can diced tomatoes (no salt added)
- One tbsp olive oil
- One tsp cumin powder
- Salt to taste

Directions:

1. Warm up your oil in a large pot on moderate temp. Add the cooked chickpeas and stir in the cumin powder for two mins.
2. Pour in the broth and diced tomatoes, then let it simmer. Let it cook for ten mins, then add the fresh spinach.
3. Cook for another five mins until the spinach is wilted. Flavor it with salt before serving.

Tips: Garnish with fresh cilantro or parsley for added flavor. Serve alongside quinoa or wild rice for a more substantial meal.

Serving size: One bowl

Nutritional values (per serving): Calories: 150; Fat: 5g; Carbs: 20g; Protein: 7g; Sodium: 300mg; Sugar: 4g; Cholesterol: 0mg; Fiber: 5g

Fresh Spring Rolls with Alkaline Dipping Sauce

Preparation time: 20 mins

Cooking time: N/A

Servings: Four

Ingredients:

- Two cups julienned carrots
- Two cups julienned cucumber
- One cup fresh mint leaves
- One cup fresh cilantro leaves
- Two cups mixed greens
- One large avocado, sliced

For the Dipping Sauce:

- Four tbsp coconut aminos
- Two tbsp lime juice
- One tsp sea salt

Directions:

1. Prepare the vegetables by washing and cutting them into thin, even slices.
2. Lay the mixed greens on a flat surface and place a small amount of each vegetable and avocado in the center.
3. Roll the greens tightly around the filling to form compact rolls.
4. To make the dipping sauce, whisk together coconut aminos, lime juice, and sea salt in a small bowl.
5. Serve the spring rolls immediately with the alkaline dipping sauce on the side.

Tips: Use any alkaline-approved vegetables you have on hand for more variety. Keep your rolls tight to avoid them falling apart.

Serving size: One roll

Nutritional values (per serving): Calories: 95; Fat: 6g; Carbs: 10g; Protein: 2g; Sodium: 320mg; Sugar: 1g; Cholesterol: 0mg; Fiber: 3g

Raw Kale and Avocado Salad

Preparation time: 15 mins

Cooking time: N/A

Servings: Four

Ingredients:

- Four cups of raw kale, chopped
- One large avocado, diced
- Two tbsp olive oil
- Three tbsp lemon juice
- One tbsp minced garlic
- Sea salt to taste

Directions:

1. In your big container, massage the chopped kale with one tablespoon of olive oil until it softens. Add the diced avocado to your container.
2. In your small container, mix remaining olive oil, lemon juice, minced garlic, and sea salt. Pour dressing over kale and avocado mixture and toss until evenly coated.

Tips: Massaging the kale reduces its bitterness and makes it easier to chew. Letting the salad sit for ten mins after dressing will enhance flavor.

Serving size: One cup

Nutritional values (per serving): Calories: 120; Fat: 11g; Carbs: 7g; Protein: 2g; Sodium: 120mg; Sugar: 0g; Cholesterol: 0mg; Fiber: 3g

Alkaline Vegetable Soup

Preparation time: 15 mins

Cooking time: 30 mins

Servings: 4

Ingredients:

- Four cups vegetable broth
- One cup chopped kale
- One cup diced zucchini
- One cup chopped green bell pepper
- One cup chopped yellow squash
- One tbsp olive oil
- Two tsp sea salt
- One tsp thyme

Directions:

1. In your big pot, warm up oil on moderate temp. Add chopped kale, zucchini, green bell pepper, and yellow squash, then sauté for five mins.
2. Pour in broth, then let it boil. Adjust to low temp, then add sea salt and thyme. Let it simmer for 25 mins, stirring occasionally. Remove, then let it cool slightly before serving.

Tips: For added flavor, garnish with fresh parsley or cilantro.

Serving size: One cup

Nutritional values (per serving): Calories: 110; Fat: 4g; Carbs: 15g; Protein: 3g; Sodium: 600mg; Sugar: 5g; Cholesterol: 0mg; Fiber: 5g

Spicy Black Bean and Sweet Potato Chili

Preparation time: 20 mins

Cooking time: 40 mins

Servings: 6

Ingredients:

- Four cups cooked black beans, canned, strained & washed
- Two cups diced sweet potatoes
- One cup diced yellow onion
- Three cups vegetable broth
- Two tbsp chili powder
- Two tsp cumin
- Three tbsp olive oil

Directions:

1. In a large pot, heat olive oil on moderate temp. Add diced yellow onion, then sauté for five mins until soft.
2. Stir in chili powder and cumin, then cook for another minute. Add diced

sweet potatoes and cook for an additional five mins.

3. Pour in broth and add black beans. Let it boil, then adjust to low temp. Let it simmer for thirty mins until sweet potatoes are tender, mixing often.
4. Remove, then let it cool slightly before serving.

Tips: Serve with a slice of lime for added zest.

Serving size: 1 cup

Nutritional values (per serving): Calories: 180; Fat: 7g; Carbs: 27g; Protein: 6g; Sodium: 500mg; Sugar: 6g; Cholesterol: 0mg; Fiber: 8g

Baked Stuffed Acorn Squash

Preparation time: 15 mins

Cooking time: 45 mins

Servings: 4

Ingredients:

- Two medium-sized acorn squash
- One cup quinoa, cooked
- Half cup chopped walnuts
- Quarter cup dried cranberries
- One tbsp olive oil
- One tsp sea salt
- Half tsp ground black pepper

Directions:

1. Warm up your oven to 400°F. Cut the acorn squash in half and scoop out the seeds.
2. Place the squash halves cut side up on a baking sheet and brush with olive oil. Sprinkle with sea salt and black pepper. Bake the squash for thirty mins until tender.
3. Meanwhile, mix cooked quinoa, walnuts, and dried cranberries in a bowl. Remove the squash, then fill each half with the quinoa mixture.
4. Place back in your oven for an additional fifteen mins until everything is heated through.

Tips: Garnish with fresh parsley or cilantro for added flavor. Use a melon baller to easily scoop out the seeds.

Serving size: Half acorn squash

Nutritional values (per serving): Calories: 190; Fat: 9g; Carbs: 26g; Protein: 5g; Sodium: 310mg; Sugar: 5g; Cholesterol: 0mg; Fiber: 4g

Garlicky Sautéed Collard Greens

Preparation time: Fifteen mins

Cooking time: Fifteen mins

Servings: Four

Ingredients:

- Two tbsp olive oil
- Four cups collard greens, chopped
- Four cloves garlic, minced
- One tsp sea salt
- One tsp black pepper

Directions:

1. Warm up oil in your big skillet on moderate temp. Add garlic and sauté for about two mins until fragrant.
2. Add collard greens and cook for about five to seven mins, stirring frequently, until wilted. Flavor it with sea salt and black pepper. Remove, then serve immediately.

Tips: Make sure the greens are completely dry before sautéing to avoid excess moisture in the pan.

Serving size: One cup

Nutritional values (per serving): Calories: 60; Fat: 4g; Carbs: 6g; Protein: 2g; Sodium: 380mg; Sugar: 1g; Cholesterol: 0mg; Fiber: 3g

Spelt Pasta with Tomato Basil Sauce

Preparation time: 10 mins

Cooking time: 20 mins

Servings: 4

Ingredients:

- Two cups spelt pasta

- Two cups cherry tomatoes, halved
- One tbsp olive oil
- Four cloves garlic, minced
- One cup fresh basil leaves, chopped
- One tsp sea salt
- One tsp black pepper

Directions:

1. Cook spelt pasta according to package instructions. Strain, then put aside. In your big pan, warm up oil on moderate temp. Add garlic, then sauté until fragrant.
2. Add cherry tomatoes, sea salt, and black pepper, then cook until tomatoes start to soften. Stir in the fresh basil leaves and cook for another two mins.
3. Add the cooked spelt pasta, then toss until pasta is well coated with the tomato basil sauce. Serve immediately.

Tips: For extra flavor, add a pinch of red pepper flakes. Use fresh tomatoes for a more vibrant taste.

Serving size: One cup

Nutritional values (per serving): Calories: 210; Fat: 5g; Carbs: 36g; Protein: 7g; Sodium: 200mg; Sugar: 3g; Cholesterol: 0mg; Fiber: 6g

Quinoa-Stuffed Bell Peppers

Preparation time: Twenty mins

Cooking time: Thirty-five mins

Servings: Four

Ingredients:

- Four bell peppers, tops removed and seeded
- One cup cooked quinoa
- One tbsp olive oil
- Two cups spinach, chopped
- One medium onion, chopped
- Two cloves garlic, minced
- One tsp cumin
- One tsp sea salt

Directions:

1. Warm up your oven to 375°F. In your big skillet, heat olive oil on moderate temp. Add onions, then sauté for five mins until translucent.
2. Add garlic and cumin, cooking for an additional two mins. Stir in spinach and cooked quinoa until well combined. Flavor it with sea salt.
3. Stuff each bell pepper with the quinoa mixture. Place stuffed peppers in a baking dish and bake for thirty-five mins or until peppers are tender.

Tips: If you prefer a spicy kick, add a pinch of red pepper flakes to the quinoa mixture.

Serving size: One stuffed pepper

Nutritional values (per serving): Calories: 150; Fat: 5g; Carbs: 22g; Protein: 4g;

Sodium: 420mg; Sugar: 4g; Cholesterol: 0mg; Fiber: 5g

Snack Recipes

Homemade Guacamole with Plantain Chips

Preparation time: 15 mins

Cooking time: 10 mins

Servings: 4

Ingredients:

- Two ripe avocados
- One tbsp lime juice
- One tsp sea salt
- One cup finely chopped cherry tomatoes
- Half cup finely chopped red onion
- Two tbsp chopped fresh cilantro
- Two large unripe plantains
- One tbsp coconut oil for frying

Directions:

1. Mash the avocados in a bowl using a fork until smooth. Add lime juice, sea salt, cherry tomatoes, red onion, and cilantro to the bowl and mix well.
2. Peel and slice plantains into thin rounds. Heat the coconut oil in a large frying pan on moderate temp.

3. Fry plantain slices until golden brown, about 2 mins per side. Remove plantain chips and let cool on a paper towel.

Tips: For added flavor, you can sprinkle a bit of sea salt over the plantain chips after frying.

Serving size: Half cup guacamole with Ten plantain chips

Nutritional values (per serving): Calories: 230; Fat: 15g; Carbs: 20g; Protein: 2g; Sodium: 300mg; Sugar: 2g; Cholesterol: 0mg; Fiber: 7g

Sautéed Zucchini and Squash Bites

Preparation time: 10 mins

Cooking time: 10 mins

Servings: 4

Ingredients:

- One lb. zucchini
- One lb. yellow squash
- Two tbsp olive oil
- One tsp sea salt
- One tsp garlic powder
- Two tbsp chopped fresh parsley or basil (optional)

Directions:

1. Wash zucchini and squash then cut into bite-sized pieces. Warm up oil

in your big pan over medium-high heat.

2. Add zucchini and squash to the pan, sprinkling with sea salt and garlic powder. Sauté for about 7-8 mins until tender but still crisp. Garnish with fresh parsley or basil if desired.

Tips: Don't overcrowd the pan to ensure even cooking.

Serving size: One cup

Nutritional values (per serving): Calories: 70; Fat: 5g; Carbs: 6g; Protein: 1g; Sodium: 250mg; Sugar: 3g; Cholesterol: 0mg; Fiber: 2g

Alkaline Kale Chips

Preparation time: 10 mins

Cooking time: 20 mins

Servings: 4

Ingredients:

- One lb. fresh kale
- Two tbsp olive oil
- One tsp sea salt
- One tsp nutritional yeast (optional for cheesy flavor)

Directions:

1. Warm up your oven to 300°F (150°C). Wash and thoroughly dry the kale leaves, then remove stems and tear into bite-sized pieces.

2. In a large bowl, drizzle olive oil over the kale and sprinkle with sea salt and nutritional yeast if using.

3. Toss until all leaves are evenly coated. Spread out kale on a baking sheet in a single layer. Bake for twenty mins until crisp, checking occasionally to ensure they do not burn.

Tips: Experiment with different seasonings like garlic powder or smoked paprika. Store chips in an airtight container to maintain crispiness.

Serving size: One cup

Nutritional values (per serving): Calories: 70; Fat: 5g; Carbs: 7g; Protein: 2g; Sodium: 240mg; Sugar: <1g; Cholesterol: 0mg; Fiber: 2g

Mango Sea Moss Smoothie Bowl

Preparation time: 10 mins

Cooking time: N/A

Servings: 2

Ingredients:

- One cup frozen mango chunks
- One tbsp sea moss gel
- One banana
- Half cup coconut water
- Half cup fresh spinach
- One tsp agave syrup (optional)

- Fresh fruits for topping (sliced kiwi, strawberries, blueberries)

Directions:

1. Add frozen mango chunks, sea moss gel, banana, coconut water, and fresh spinach to a blender. Blend until smooth and creamy.
2. Pour the smoothie into two bowls. Top with sliced fresh fruits and a drizzle of agave syrup if using.

Tips: For added crunch, add a sprinkle of chia seeds or granola. Change the toppings to your liking for variety.

Serving size: 1 bowl

Nutritional values (per serving): Calories: 150; Fat: 1g; Carbs: 35g; Protein: 2g; Sodium: 20mg; Sugar: 20g; Cholesterol: 0mg; Fiber: 5g

Electric Fruit Salad with Berries and Melons

Preparation time: 15 mins

Cooking time: N/A

Servings: 4

Ingredients:

- Two cups watermelon, cubed
- One cup cantaloupe, cubed
- One cup strawberries, hulled and sliced
- One cup blueberries

- Juice of one lime
- One tbsp raw agave nectar

Directions:

1. In a large bowl, combine watermelon, cantaloupe, strawberries, and blueberries.
2. Drizzle lime juice and raw agave nectar over the mixed fruits. Gently toss all ingredients until evenly coated.

Tips: Serve chilled for a refreshing experience. You can sprinkle some mint leaves for an extra burst of flavor.

Serving size: One cup

Nutritional values (per serving): Calories: 90; Fat: 0g; Carbs: 23g; Protein: 1g; Sodium: 10mg; Sugar: 18g; Cholesterol: 0mg; Fiber: 4g

Dr. Sebi's Approved Trail Seeds Mix

Preparation time: 5 mins

Cooking time: N/A

Servings: 4

Ingredients:

- One cup raw pumpkin seeds
- One cup raw sunflower seeds
- One-third cup sesame seeds
- One-fourth cup hemp seeds

Directions:

1. In a large mixing bowl, combine all the seeds.
2. Stir well to ensure an even mix. Store in an airtight container.

Tips: Add a dash of sea salt if you prefer a salty snack. You can sprinkle this mix on salads or smoothies for added crunch and nutrition.

Serving size: Quarter cup

Nutritional values (per serving): Calories: 210; Fat: 18g; Carbs: 8g; Protein: 9g; Sodium: 0mg; Sugar: 1g; Cholesterol: 0mg; Fiber: 4g

Spelt Flour Crackers with Hummus

Preparation time: 15 mins

Cooking time: 20 mins

Servings: 6

Ingredients:

- One & half cups of spelt flour
- Half tsp sea salt
- Three tbsp olive oil
- Half cup water

For the Hummus:

- One and one-fourth cups of cooked chickpeas
- Three tbsp tahini
- Two tbsp lemon juice
- One garlic clove, minced
- Three tbsp olive oil
- Half tsp sea salt

Directions:

1. Warm up your oven to 350°F. In your container, mix spelt flour and sea salt. Add olive oil and water, mixing until dough forms.
2. Roll the dough out on a floured surface to about one-eighth inch thickness. Cut into desired shapes and place on a baking sheet lined with parchment paper.
3. Bake for fifteen to twenty mins or until golden brown. In a food processor, combine chickpeas, tahini, lemon juice, garlic, olive oil, and sea salt. Blend until smooth.
4. If you prefer thinner hummus, add water one tablespoon at a time until desired consistency is reached.

Tips: Store crackers in an airtight container to keep them crisp. Garnish hummus with a drizzle of olive oil and paprika before serving.

Serving size: Two crackers with two tbsp hummus

Nutritional values (per serving): Calories: 180; Fat: 10g; Carbs: 20g; Protein: 4g; Sodium: 200mg; Sugar: 1g; Cholesterol: 0mg; Fiber: 3g

Spicy Okra Chips

Preparation time: 10 mins

Cooking time: 25 mins

Servings: 4

Ingredients:

- One lb. fresh okra
- One tbsp olive oil
- One tsp cayenne pepper
- One tsp sea salt
- One tsp smoked paprika

Directions:

1. Warm up your oven to 400°F (200°C). Wash and pat dry the okra, then slice them lengthwise.
2. In your big container, toss the okra slices with olive oil, cayenne pepper, sea salt, and smoked paprika until evenly coated.
3. Spread the okra slices out on a baking sheet. Bake in the preheated oven for about 20-25 mins or until they are crispy, turning them halfway through.
4. Remove, then allow to cool for a few mins before serving.

Tips: For even crispier chips, try using a wire rack on top of your baking sheet to allow air circulation underneath the okra slices. Adjust spice levels according to your preference.

Serving size: One cup

Nutritional values (per serving): Calories: 90; Fat: 6g; Carbs: 8g; Protein: 2g; Sodium: 240mg; Sugar: 1g; Cholesterol: 0mg; Fiber: 4g

Dr. Sebi's Approved Fruit Popsicles

Preparation time: 10 mins + freezing time

Cooking time: N/A

Servings: 6

Ingredients:

- Two cups fresh berries (such as strawberries, blueberries, raspberries)
- One cup coconut water
- Two tbsp agave syrup
- One tsp lime juice

Directions:

1. Wash and hull the berries. Combine the berries, coconut water, agave syrup, and lime juice in a blender. Blend until smooth.
2. Pour the mixture into popsicle molds. Freeze for four hours or until completely solid.

Tips: Use fresh, ripe fruits for the best flavor. You can mix different berries for a varied taste.

Serving size: One popsicle

Nutritional values (per serving): Calories: 50; Fat: 0g; Carbs: 13g; Protein: 0g; Sodium: 5mg; Sugar: 11g; Cholesterol: 0mg; Fiber: 2g

Burro Banana and Nut Butter Bites

Preparation time: 10 mins

Cooking time: N/A

Servings: 12 bites

Ingredients:

- Three burro bananas (ripe)
- Half cup raw almond butter
- One tbsp shredded unsweetened coconut
- One tsp cinnamon powder
- One tbsp agave syrup

Directions:

1. Peel and slice the burro bananas into thick rounds. Spread almond butter on top of each banana slice.
2. Sprinkle shredded coconut and cinnamon powder over each piece. Drizzle with agave syrup for added sweetness.

Tips: Serve immediately for freshness. Can be refrigerated for a cooler snack.

Serving size: Two bites

Nutritional values (per serving): Calories: 90; Fat: 4g; Carbs: 14g; Protein: 2g; Sodium: 0mg; Sugar: 7g; Cholesterol: 0mg; Fiber: 3g

Meal Plans That Cater to Different Dietary Needs and Restrictions

From allergies to intolerances, to specific dietary choices and medical conditions, creating meal plans that cater to these needs is not only beneficial but necessary for overall health and well-being. When planning meals for different dietary needs, variety is key. Incorporating the right balance of nutrients while adhering to restrictions can be a challenge, but with thoughtful planning, it's entirely manageable. Let's explore some common dietary requirements and how you can tailor your meal plans accordingly.

Gluten-Free Diet Meal Plan

For those with celiac disease or gluten sensitivity, avoiding gluten is crucial. Fortunately, there are plenty of options without gluten that are both nutritious and delicious. Many grains such as quinoa, teff, and wild rice can easily replace gluten-containing grains like wheat. Breakfast could include *Quinoa Porridge with Fresh Berries* or *Teff Pancakes with Agave Syrup*.

For lunch or dinner, *Spelt Pasta with Tomato Basil Sauce* can be substituted with quinoa pasta or any gluten-free alternative. Snacks like *Spelt Flour Crackers* might need tweaking, but Sautéed *Zucchini and Squash Bites* make a perfect substitute.

DAY	BREAKFAST	LUNCH	SNACK	DINNER
1	Quinoa Porridge with Fresh Berries	Quinoa Pasta with Tomato Basil Sauce	Sautéed Zucchini and Squash Bites	Grilled Portobello Mushrooms with Herbs
2	Apple-Cinnamon Quinoa Breakfast Bake	Wild Rice and Bell Pepper Stir-Fry	Dr. Sebi's Approved Fruit Popsicles	Zucchini Noodles with Tahini Sauce
3	Soursop Smoothie with Chia Seeds	Cauliflower Rice with Tempeh Stir-fry	Alkaline Kale Chips	Chickpea and Spinach Stew
4	Butternut Squash Hash Browns	Spicy Lentil Soup with Cayenne Pepper	Mango Sea Moss Smoothie Bowl	Spicy Black Bean and Sweet Potato Chili
5	Teff Pancakes with Agave Syrup	Roasted Garlic and Tomato Soup	Dr. Sebi's Approved Trail Seeds Mix	Baked Stuffed Acorn Squash

6	Chia Seed Pudding with Agave Syrup	Portobello Mushroom Burgers	Spicy Okra Chips	Fresh Spring Rolls with Alkaline Dipping Sauce
7	Sea Moss and Bladderwrack Smoothie	Raw Kale and Avocado Salad	Electric Fruit Salad with Berries and Melons	Quinoa-Stuffed Bell Peppers

Vegan Diet Meal Plan

A vegan diet excludes all animal products, focusing entirely on plant-based foods. This aligns well with Dr. Sebi's nutritional guide which emphasizes plant-based eating. Dishes like *Cauliflower Rice with Tempeh Stir-fry* or *Chickpea and Spinach Stew* serve as excellent lunch or dinner choices. For breakfast, *Chia Seed Pudding with Agave Syrup* offers a creamy, nutrient-packed start to the day without animal products.

DAY	BREAKFAST	LUNCH	SNACK	DINNER
1	Dr. Sebi's Banana Walnut Bread	Bell Pepper and Avocado Wraps	Homemade Guacamole with Plantain Chips	Alkaline Vegetable Soup
2	Alkaline Green Power Juice	Butternut Squash Soup with Ginger	Spelt Flour Crackers with Hummus	Garlicky Sautéed Collard Greens
3	Spelt Flour Banana Muffins	Sautéed Zucchini and Squash Medley	Burro Banana and Nut Butter Bites	Zucchini Noodles with Tahini Sauce
4	Sea Moss and Bladderwrack Smoothie	Cauliflower Rice with Tempeh Stir-fry	Dr. Sebi's Approved Fruit Popsicles	Fresh Spring Rolls with Alkaline Dipping Sauce
5	Teff Pancakes with Agave Syrup	Wild Rice and Bell Pepper Stir-Fry	Mango Sea Moss Smoothie Bowl	Spicy Black Bean and Sweet Potato Chili
6	Chia Seed Pudding with Agave Syrup	Roasted Garlic and Tomato Soup	Electric Fruit Salad with Berries and Melons	Quinoa-Stuffed Bell Peppers
7	Butternut Squash	Portobello Mushroom	Dr. Sebi's Approved Trail	Chickpea and

| | Hash Browns | Burgers | Seeds Mix | Spinach Stew |

Nut-Free Diet Meal Plan

Nuts are a common allergen that many individuals must avoid. Ensuring meals are free from nuts requires vigilance but isn't difficult within Dr. Sebi's framework. For instance, the *Banana Walnut Bread* recipe can be made nut-free by omitting walnuts or substituting them with seeds such as pumpkin seeds or sunflower seeds. Similarly, snacks like Burro Banana and Nut Butter Bites can be modified by using seed butter instead of nut butter.

DAY	BREAKFAST	LUNCH	SNACK	DINNER
1	Quinoa Porridge with Fresh Berries	Bell Pepper and Avocado Wraps	Mango Sea Moss Smoothie Bowl	Alkaline Vegetable Soup
2	Apple-Cinnamon Quinoa Breakfast Bake	Roasted Garlic and Tomato Soup	Electric Fruit Salad with Berries and Melons	Zucchini Noodles with Tahini Sauce
3	Soursop Smoothie with Chia Seeds	Cauliflower Rice with Tempeh Stir-fry	Dr. Sebi's Approved Fruit Popsicles	Spicy Lentil Soup with Cayenne Pepper
4	Chia Seed Pudding with Agave Syrup	Portobello Mushroom Burgers	Alkaline Kale Chips	Baked Stuffed Acorn Squash
5	Teff Pancakes with Agave Syrup	Grilled Portobello Mushrooms with Herbs	Spelt Flour Crackers with Hummus	Garlicky Sautéed Collard Greens
6	Butternut Squash Hash Browns	Wild Rice and Bell Pepper Stir-Fry	Dr. Sebi's Approved Trail Seeds Mix	Chickpea and Spinach Stew
7	Sea Moss and Bladderwrack Smoothie	Sautéed Zucchini and Squash Medley	Homemade Guacamole with Plantain Chips	Quinoa-Stuffed Bell Peppers

Low-Sugar Diet Meal Plan

Some individuals need to monitor their sugar intake due to conditions like diabetes or just as a personal health choice. Reducing sugar does not mean compromising on taste or nutrition.

Smoothies like *Soursop Smoothie with Chia Seeds* serve as an excellent option because they use natural sweetness from fruits.

Additionally, recipes like *Alkaline Green Power Juice* provide lots of nutrients without the high sugar content you'll find in many commercial beverages.

DAY	BREAKFAST	LUNCH	SNACK	DINNER
1	Chia Seed Pudding (sugar-free version)	Grilled Portobello Mushrooms with Herbs	Alkaline Kale Chips	Zucchini Noodles with Tahini Sauce
2	Sea Moss and Bladderwrack Smoothie (without sweeteners)	Cauliflower Rice with Tempeh Stir-fry	Spicy Okra Chips	Fresh Spring Rolls with Alkaline Dipping Sauce
3	Butternut Squash Hash Browns	Butternut Squash Soup with Ginger (no added sugars)	Sautéed Zucchini and Squash Bites	Chickpea and Spinach Stew
4	Alkaline Green Power Juice (sugar-free)	Raw Kale and Avocado Salad	Dr. Sebi's Approved Trail Seeds Mix	Spicy Black Bean and Sweet Potato Chili (no sugar)
5	Teff Pancakes with Agave Syrup (minimal syrup)	Wild Rice and Bell Pepper Stir-Fry	Electric Fruit Salad with Berries and Melons (no sweeteners)	Garlicky Sautéed Collard Greens
6	Soursop Smoothie with Chia Seeds (unsweetened)	Bell Pepper and Avocado Wraps	Dr. Sebi's Approved Fruit Popsicles	Quinoa-Stuffed Bell Peppers
7	Spelt Flour Banana Muffins (no sweetener)	Roasted Garlic & Tomato Soup (sugar-free version)	Mango Sea Moss Smoothie Bowl (sugar free)	Spelt Pasta With Tomato Basil sauce (no sugar)

High-Protein Diet Meal Plan

High-protein diets are often sought after by those looking to build muscle or manage their weight effectively. While Dr. Sebi's diet mainly focuses on alkaline foods which may be lower in protein compared to conventional diets rich in animal products, there are good plant-based sources of protein such as legumes and certain grains.

Consider meals such as *Lentil Soup with Cayenne Pepper* for lunch and *Grilled Portobello Mushrooms* for dinner—these provide substantial protein sources from plants.

DAY	BREAKFAST	LUNCH	SNACK	DINNER
1	Quinoa Porridge with Fresh Berries	Portobello Mushroom Burgers	Homemade Guacamole with Plantain Chips	Chickpea and Spinach Stew
2	Soursop Smoothie with Chia Seeds	Spicy Lentil Soup with Cayenne Pepper	Mango Sea Moss Smoothie Bowl	Baked Stuffed Acorn Squash
3	Apple-Cinnamon Quinoa Breakfast Bake	Grilled Portobello Mushrooms with Herbs	Sautéed Zucchini and Squash Bites	Spelt Pasta with Tomato Basil Sauce
4	Chia Seed Pudding with Agave Syrup	Raw Kale and Avocado Salad	Electric Fruit Salad with Berries and Melons	Alkaline Vegetable Soup
5	Teff Pancakes with Agave Syrup	Cauliflower Rice with Tempeh Stir-fry	Dr. Sebi's Approved Trail Seeds Mix	Fresh Spring Rolls with Alkaline Dipping Sauce
6	Dr. Sebi's Banana Walnut Bread	Wild Rice and Bell Pepper Stir-Fry	Spicy Okra Chips	Spicy Black Bean and Sweet Potato Chili
7	Quinoa Porridge with Fresh Berries	Roasted Garlic and Tomato Soup	Dr. Sebi's Approved Fruit Popsicles	Garlicky Sautéed Collard Greens

Advice on Meal Preparation and Maintaining Nutritional Balance

Maintaining nutritional balance while following the principles of Dr. Sebi's Mucus Cleanse is crucial. As someone who has embarked on this journey, I understand that meal preparation can seem daunting at first. However, with the right advice and a clear routine, it becomes much easier and beneficial to your health.

The first step in effective meal preparation is understanding which foods are allowed. Dr. Sebi's diet focuses heavily on natural, alkaline foods that help the body maintain a balanced pH level. This includes a variety of fruits, vegetables, nuts, seeds, grains like quinoa and spelt, and herbal teas. Here are some tips for meal preparation:

1. **Plan Your Meals in Advance:** Start by planning your meals for the week. Write down your breakfast, lunch, dinner, and snacks for each day. This will not only save you time but also ensure you have all the necessary ingredients.
2. **Grocery Shopping:** Once you have a meal plan, create a shopping list based on the ingredients you need. Stick to this list to avoid purchasing non-compliant foods.
3. **Batch Cooking:** Cooking in bulk can save you time and help you stick to your nutritional goals. Choose a day, usually at the start of the week, to prepare several meals that can be stored in the refrigerator or freezer.
4. **Storage:** Invest in good quality storage containers that keep food fresh longer. Glass containers are preferable as they do not leach chemicals into food.
5. **Keep it Simple:** Start with simple recipes that require minimal ingredients and steps. This reduces stress and makes meal prep manageable.

Maintaining Nutritional Balance

Dr. Sebi's diet emphasizes a balance of essential nutrients such as vitamins, minerals, proteins, fats, and carbohydrates derived from plant-based sources. To maintain nutritional balance:

1. **Fruit Variety:** Incorporate a variety of fruits into your diet including berries, apples, grapes, oranges, and watermelons. These provide essential vitamins such as Vitamin C and antioxidants.
2. **Vegetable Diversity:** Vary your vegetable intake with options like kale, spinach, cucumber, bell peppers, zucchini, and tomatoes. These vegetables supply essential minerals such as iron (from leafy greens) and magnesium.
3. **Healthy Fats:** Include healthy fats from sources like avocados, coconut oil or hemp seeds which are crucial for brain function and hormone production.
4. **Complex Carbohydrates:** Foods such as quinoa and spelt flour not only keep you satiated but are rich in protein and other nutrients important for energy production.

5. **Proteins**: Incorporate plant-based proteins like chickpeas and nuts into your meals to ensure you get adequate protein intake without resorting to animal products.

Drinking enough water is essential. Aim for at least 8 glasses of spring water each day. You can also enjoy herbal teas made from approved herbs like burdock root, nettle, and red raspberry. Pay attention to how your body responds to different foods. Everyone's body is unique, and learning what works for you is important. If certain foods make you feel energized, make sure to include them in your diet regularly.

Tracking Your Nutritional Intake

Creating a simple chart can help you monitor your nutritional intake and ensure you're getting a balanced diet. Here's an example of how you could structure it:

FOOD GROUP	EXAMPLE FOODS	TARGET INTAKE
Fruits	Berries, apples, grapes	3-4 servings per day
Vegetables	Kale, spinach, zucchini	4-5 servings per day
Healthy Fats	Avocado, hemp seeds	2-3 tablespoons of healthy fats per day
Complex Carbs	Quinoa, spelt flour products	Include in 2 meals per day
Proteins	Chickpeas, nuts	2 servings of plant-based proteins per day

Helpful Tips

1. **Stay Organized:** Keep your kitchen well-organized so that meal preparation and cooking are smooth processes. Label containers with names and dates.
2. **Hydration:** Besides drinking water, eating fruits with high water content like watermelon helps keep you hydrated.
3. **Seasonal Eating:** Try to eat fruits and vegetables that are in season for the best nutrition and taste experience.

By sticking to these guidelines, meal preparation will be less stressful, and maintaining nutritional balance on Dr. Sebi's Mucus Cleanse will become second nature. Remember, this journey is about creating sustainable habits that support long-term health.

CHAPTER 6

Integrating the Cleanse into Everyday Life

Strategies for Making Dr. Sebi's Methods a Sustainable Part of Daily Routines

Developing a sustainable routine around Dr. Sebi's methods involves integrating his principles into our daily lives in a way that feels seamless and natural. Here are some strategies to make this possible:

1. **Embrace Simplicity in Meal Planning**: One of the easiest ways to make Dr. Sebi's methods sustainable is by simplifying your meal planning. Focus on a core set of alkaline foods that you enjoy and that are readily available in your area. Rotate these foods throughout the week to keep things interesting but manageable. For instance, you can start your day with a smoothie made from fresh fruits like berries and alkaline greens, followed by a hearty salad with mixed vegetables for lunch, and finish with a nourishing vegetable soup or stir-fry for dinner.

2. **Batch Cooking and Meal Prepping**: Batch cooking is an excellent way to ensure you always have healthy meals ready to go, even on your busiest days. Spend a couple of hours once or twice a week preparing large quantities of grains, legumes, and vegetables. Store them in portion-sized containers so you can quickly assemble meals throughout the week. This approach minimizes the need for last-minute unhealthy choices.

3. **Incorporate Dr. Sebi-Approved Snacks**: Snacking smartly is key to maintaining energy levels and staying on track with Dr. Sebi's methods. Keep your pantry stocked with approved snacks like nuts, seeds, fresh fruits, and homemade veggie chips. This way, you'll always have something nutritious to grab when hunger strikes between meals.

4. **Create Personalized Herbal Remedies**: Herbs play a crucial role in Dr. Sebi's approach to health. Instead of relying solely on store-bought supplements, learn how to create your

herbal remedies using fresh herbs at home. For example, prepare herbal teas using ingredients like burdock root or chamomile that support cleansing and overall health.

5. **Monitor Your Progress**: Tracking your progress can be incredibly motivating and provide insights into what works best for you. Keep a journal where you note down what you eat, how it makes you feel, and any changes in your health or energy levels. Regularly reviewing this can help you stay committed to the routine and make necessary adjustments along the way.

6. **Mindful Eating Practices**: Mindful eating involves paying close attention to what you're eating and how it makes you feel, both physically and emotionally. It's about slowing down, savoring each bite, and being present during meals. This practice can help reinforce positive habits associated with Dr. Sebi's diet while helping you tune into your body's needs more effectively.

7. **Find Like-Minded Community Support**: Connecting with others who follow Dr. Sebi's methods can provide invaluable support and motivation. Join local or online communities where you can share experiences, exchange recipes, and encourage each other through challenges. Being part of a community can also provide practical tips and emotional reinforcement that make sustaining these practices easier.

8. **Continuous Learning**: Health is a journey rather than a destination; therefore, continually educating yourself about holistic health practices can keep your motivation high. Read books on natural healing, attend seminars or workshops related to Dr. Sebi's teachings, or follow reputable blogs and social media accounts dedicated to alkaline living.

9. **Integrate Exercise Regularly**: Physical activity complements dietary changes beautifully by enhancing circulation and aiding detoxification processes described by Dr. Sebi's regimen. Incorporate moderate exercise such as walking, yoga, or swimming into daily routines—not only does this boost overall health but it also supports metabolic processes essential for cleansing.

10. **Creating Rituals Around Food Preparation**: Turn meal preparation from a chore into an enjoyable ritual by involving all senses—select vibrant vegetables mindfully; listen to soothing music while cooking; and take the time to appreciate the aromas of the ingredients as they cook. By making meal prep an enjoyable activity rather than a task, you'll be more likely to stick with Dr. Sebi's dietary recommendations over time.

11. **Routine Detoxification Practices**: Regular detoxification is essential in maintaining the benefits of Dr. Sebi's methods. Incorporate simple detox practices into your routine, such as drinking warm lemon water each morning or taking detox baths with Epsom salts and baking soda. These small habits can aid in cleansing the body and promoting overall health.

12. **Mind-Body Connection**: Understanding and strengthening the mind-body connection can further support the sustainability of Dr. Sebi's methods. Practices like meditation, deep breathing exercises, and mindfulness can reduce stress and improve mental clarity, making it easier to adhere to your routines.

13. **Family Involvement**: Getting your family involved in Dr. Sebi's way of eating can make it more enjoyable and sustainable. Prepare meals together, educate them on the benefits of alkaline foods, and involve them in grocery shopping. When everyone is on board, creating a daily routine around these principles becomes much more manageable.

14. **Adapting Recipes to Fit Your Lifestyle**: Flexibility is key to sustainability. Adapt traditional recipes to fit Dr. Sebi's guidelines without compromising on flavor or satisfaction. For example, you can replace wheat flour with spelt flour in baked goods or use zucchini noodles instead of pasta.

Incorporating these strategies into your daily life can make Dr. Sebi's methods a long-term lifestyle rather than a temporary diet. With consistent effort and mindful practices, you can enjoy lasting health benefits.

STRATEGY	ACTION STEPS
Embrace Simplicity	Simplify meal plans using core alkaline foods
Batch Cooking	Prepare large quantities of grains, legumes, vegetables
Snacks	Stock approved snacks like nuts, seeds, fruits
Herbal Remedies	Create herbal teas from fresh herbs
Monitor Progress	Keep a journal of meals and health changes
Mindful Eating	Focus on eating slowly and being present
Community Support	Join groups for motivation and shared experiences
Continuous Learning	Read books and attend seminars on holistic health
Exercise	Incorporate walking or yoga into daily routine
Enjoyable Meal Prep	Make cooking a sensory-rich, enjoyable activity

Detox Practices	Add simple detox habits like lemon water in mornings
Mind-Body Practices	Practice meditation and deep breathing exercises
Family Involvement	Cook together and educate family members
Recipe Adaptation	Modify traditional recipes for alkaline compliance

Tips For Dining Out, Traveling, And Managing Social Occasions

Eating out, traveling, and handling social situations can be challenging when you're committed to a mucus cleanse. With a bit of planning and mindfulness, you can navigate these situations without compromising your health goals. Here are practical tips to help you stay on track.

Dining Out

1. **Research Ahead:** Before heading out to a restaurant, look up the menu online. Most establishments have their menus available on their websites. This allows you to find mucus-friendly options ahead of time.
2. **Ask Questions:** Don't hesitate to ask your server about ingredients and preparation methods. Explain that you have dietary restrictions and need details on how dishes are prepared.
3. **Customize Orders:** Most restaurants are happy to accommodate special requests. Ask for grilled or steamed vegetables instead of fried sides, or request sauces and dressings on the side.
4. **Salads Are Your Friend:** Salads can be an excellent option if you ensure they are made with fresh, mucus-free ingredients. Opt for oil and vinegar dressings rather than creamy ones.
5. **Avoid Hidden Mucus-Causing Ingredients:** Things like dairy, white flour, and processed sugars often sneak into dishes. Learn to spot these on menus and avoid them.

Traveling

1. **Pack Snacks:** One way to stay on track while traveling is bringing your own snacks. Pack easy-to-carry items like nuts, seeds, fresh fruit, or homemade vegetable chips.
2. **Stay Hydrated:** Traveling can quickly lead to dehydration, which can increase mucus production. Carry a water bottle with you and drink plenty of water throughout the day.

3. **Plan Ahead:** Look up grocery stores and health food shops around your travel destination where you can buy fresh produce and other healthy options.

4. **Choose Accommodations Wisely:** Consider staying somewhere with kitchen facilities so you can prepare some of your meals instead of relying solely on restaurants.

5. **Air Travel Tips:** If you're flying, airport food can be a challenge. Bring your own prepared meals or check the airport's website for healthier dining options available in the terminals.

Managing Social Occasions

1. **Offer to Bring Your Own Dish:** If you're attending a potluck or family gathering, offer to bring a dish that fits within your dietary plan. This ensures there is at least one mucus-free option available for you to enjoy.

2. **Communicate Your Needs:** Be open with friends and family about your dietary choices ahead of time so they understand your needs and potential challenges during meals together.

3. **Eat Beforehand: If** you're unsure about the available food options at an event, have a small meal before you go so that you're not too hungry once there.

4. **Focus on the Company, Not Just Food:** Social occasions are as much about enjoying the company as they are about eating. Engage in conversations, play games, or take part in activities that shift attention away from food-centered discussions.

5. **Stay Positive and Flexible:** Remember that maintaining a mucus cleanse is a personal journey. Don't stress if once in a while things don't go as planned; what's important is making consistent efforts toward better health.

How to Adapt the Principles for Families, Including Children and Elderly

Maintaining a healthy diet is essential at all ages, but the approach may vary based on the different needs of family members. One major aspect of Dr. Sebi's principles is consuming alkaline foods. For families, it is crucial to design a meal plan that everyone can enjoy without feeling restricted.

Breakfast Ideas

For breakfast, start with simple yet nutritious options. Smoothies packed with fruits like berries and bananas are a hit with kids. Add some chia seeds or kale to boost nutrition without altering the taste much. Whole-grain cereals with almond or coconut milk can also be a good choice. For elderly family members, soft and easily digestible foods like oatmeal flavored with a drizzle of agave nectar and fresh fruit will be gentle on the digestive system.

Lunch and Dinner

Lunch should be light but satisfying. Salads packed with leafy greens like spinach and arugula, topped with grilled vegetables such as bell peppers and zucchini, can keep energy levels stable throughout the day. Use dressings made from lime juice, avocado oil, or apple cider vinegar to add flavor without resorting to processed options.

Dinner can include more substantial meals like vegetable stir-fries or soups made from approved ingredients such as squash, okra, or chickpeas. Remember to use natural herbs like basil and thyme instead of salt-heavy seasonings.

Snacks

Healthy snacking is crucial in preventing unhealthy cravings. Keep a bowl of cut-up fruits like mangoes and apples available at all times. Nuts such as almonds and walnuts can serve as excellent snack options as well.

Getting Kids on Board

Children are naturally resistant to change when it comes to diet, so making the transition fun and engaging is vital.

1. **Make It Interactive:** Involve kids in preparing their meals. Allow them to pick out fruits for their smoothies or garnish their salads with nuts and seeds they choose themselves. The more they contribute, the more likely they are to enjoy what they eat.
2. **Education Through Fun:** Teach kids about nutrition through fun activities such as colorful charts showing which foods are "superfoods." You can even turn it into a game where they earn points for eating these foods daily.
3. **Consistency:** Introduce new foods gradually. Start by replacing one meal per day with an alkaline meal and gradually increase this until most meals follow Dr. Sebi's principles.

Catering to the Elderly

The elderly often have special dietary requirements due to age-related health issues like reduced metabolism or dental problems.

1. **Ease of Digestion:** Focus on foods that are easy to digest yet packed with nutrients. Soups and stews made from root vegetables like carrots and sweet potatoes can be comforting and easy on the stomach while providing much-needed vitamins and minerals.

2. **Soft Textures:** Opt for softer foods that don't require much chewing. Mashed avocados make an excellent addition to toast or salads for added healthy fats without requiring extensive chewing.

3. **Hydration:** Elderly individuals often face issues related to dehydration due to decreased sense of thirst. Include hydrating foods like cucumbers, watermelon, and oranges in their diet to keep them hydrated effortlessly.

4. **Monitoring Progress:** Maintaining a food journal can help track what works best for each family member. Note down which meals each person enjoys most and any changes in health observed over time.

FAMILY MEMBER	FAVORITE MEALS	HEALTH CHANGES OBSERVED
Mom	Fruit Smoothies	Increased energy, fewer cravings
Dad	Vegetable stir-fries	Weight loss, improved digestion
Grandma	Oatmeal with fruits	Better digestion, more energy
Grandpa	Soups and stews with root vegetables	Easier digestion, better hydration
Daughter	Whole-grain cereals with almond milk	More focused in school
Son	Mango and apple slices	Happier mood, no afternoon slumps

Maintaining a routine where everyone eats together can build a sense of community and make it easier to stick to the plan. Have set meal times and involve everyone in meal preparation. Praise family members for sticking to their healthy meals. Little celebrations like movie nights or outdoor activities can keep everyone motivated.

By making small but meaningful adjustments to Dr. Sebi's principles, it's entirely possible to create a family-inclusive approach that benefits everyone. From engaging kids in meal prep to ensuring elderly members get soft, nutrient-rich foods, this lifestyle can adapt to each person's needs effectively. Keeping a close eye on everyone's preferences and health outcomes ensures the journey is enjoyable and sustainable for the whole family.

CHAPTER 7

Overcoming Challenges and Staying on Track

Common Challenges Readers May Face and Practical Solutions

When you're embarking on a journey like Dr. Sebi's Mucus Cleanse, it's normal to encounter a few bumps in the road. Here, we'll explore some common challenges and practical solutions to help you stay on track.

Challenge 1: Adapting to a New Diet

Changing your diet significantly can be hard. If you're not used to eating plant-based foods or avoiding certain ingredients, it can feel overwhelming.

Solution: Start slowly. Gradually eliminate foods that are not part of Dr. Sebi's plan. Introduce one or two new foods each week to make the transition smoother. Planning meals in advance can also help you stay organized.

Challenge 2: Cravings for Old Foods

Old habits die hard, especially when it comes to food cravings. Craving for sugar, caffeine, or processed foods can be intense when starting the cleanse.

Solution: Whenever cravings hit, try to find healthier alternatives that fit within Dr. Sebi's guidelines. For instance, if you crave something sweet, opt for fruits like dates or figs. Drink herbal teas instead of coffee to satisfy your caffeine needs.

Challenge 3: Social Situations

Social events often involve food that may not align with your new dietary choices.

Solution: Be proactive and communicate your needs ahead of time. Inform your friends or family about your dietary restrictions so they can offer suitable options or let you bring your own dishes.

Challenge 4: Availability of Ingredients

Sometimes finding specific ingredients recommended by Dr. Sebi can be a challenge.

Solution: Online stores are a great resource for hard-to-find items. Also, make use of local health food stores which might carry the ingredients you need. Don't hesitate to ask store managers if they can stock certain products for you.

Challenge 5: Initial Detox Symptoms

When starting the cleanse, some people experience detox symptoms like headaches, fatigue, or irritability as their body adjusts.

Solution: Stay hydrated and get plenty of rest during this period. Drinking alkaline water and herbal teas can help alleviate some symptoms. Ensure you're consuming enough calories to fuel your body throughout the day.

Challenge 6: Managing Time for Meal Prep

Adhering to a mostly raw food diet requires significant meal prep time, which can be challenging if you have a busy schedule.

Solution: Dedicate a few hours once a week for meal prep. Prepare large batches of ingredients and store them in portion sizes so they're ready when you need them. Invest in good kitchen tools like a high-quality blender and food processor to make prep easier.

CHALLENGE	SOLUTION
Adapting to a New Diet	Start slowly; plan meals in advance
Cravings for Old Foods	Find healthier alternatives
Social Situations	Communicate dietary needs; bring your own dish
Availability of Ingredients	Use online stores; ask local shop managers
Initial Detox Symptoms	Stay hydrated; get plenty of rest; drink herbal teas
Managing Time for Meal Prep	Dedicate weekly meal prep time; prepare large batches

Undertaking Dr. Sebi's Mucus Cleanse is no small feat but being aware of these common challenges allows us to tackle them head-on with practical solutions. Remember that every step forward is progress towards better health!

Handling Setbacks and Maintaining Long-Term Health Improvements

The path to long-term health improvements is rarely a straight line. Whether it's indulging in unhealthy foods, missing a few days of exercise, or feeling overwhelmed by stress, everyone experiences moments where they deviate from their health plans. The key is not to let these setbacks define you or derail your progress.

One effective way to handle setbacks is by adopting a growth mindset. A growth mindset revolves around the belief that challenges and failures are opportunities for growth and learning. Instead of viewing a setback as a failure, see it as a chance to understand yourself better and make necessary adjustments. For example, if you slip up on your diet, don't chastise yourself; instead, analyze what led to the slip-up. Were you stressed? Were healthy options unavailable? Use this insight to prepare better in the future.

Another crucial aspect of handling setbacks is self-compassion. Be kind to yourself during these times. Remember that self-criticism can often lead to further setbacks, whereas self-compassion fosters resilience. Reflect on how far you've come and remind yourself of your long-term goals. Encourage yourself just like you would encourage a close friend.

Having a support network can also make a significant difference when dealing with setbacks. Surround yourself with individuals who understand your goals and can offer support and encouragement during tough times. This could be family members, friends, or even online communities focused on health improvement. Sharing your experiences with others can provide motivation and accountability.

In addition to mental strategies, practical tools can help prevent future setbacks:

1. **Meal Planning:** Plan your meals ahead of time to ensure you have healthy options available, reducing the temptation to resort to unhealthy food choices.
2. **Exercise Routine:** Establishing a consistent exercise routine helps make physical activity a regular part of your day.
3. **Stress Management:** Incorporate stress-relief practices such as meditation, deep breathing exercises, or yoga into your daily routine.
4. **Sleep Hygiene:** Ensure you're getting adequate sleep each night as poor sleep can negatively impact both your physical health and decision-making abilities.

To maintain long-term health improvements, tracking your progress is essential. Keeping a journal or using an app can help you monitor what works well for you and what doesn't. Note down any patterns you observe during setbacks so that you can proactively address them in the future.

Here's a simple table format you can use in your journal:

DATE	SETBACK EXPERIENCED	Possible Cause	ACTION TAKEN	REFLECTION/OUT COME
MM/DD/YYYY	Missed workout	Lack of time	Scheduled shorter session	Felt more accomplished
MM/DD/YYYY	Ate junk food	High stress	Practiced meditation	Reduced stress levels
MM/DD/YYYY	Skipped meal prep	Poor planning	Prepped on weekend	Availability of healthy meals

Consistency doesn't mean perfection; it means continuously striving towards improvement despite occasional missteps. Take each day as an opportunity for betterment rather than focusing solely on the end goal.

Remember that long-term health improvements are cumulative and incremental. Small daily actions contribute significantly over time to overall well-being. Celebrate small victories along the way—whether it's choosing a healthy snack over junk food or completing an extra 10 mins of exercise. Acknowledge these successes as building blocks towards your ultimate health goals.

Another important point is to diversify your health activities. Prevent monotony by trying new recipes, different types of physical activities, or new stress-relief techniques. Variety keeps you engaged and can help you discover methods that you enjoy more and are less likely to abandon.

HEALTHY ACTIVITIES	BENEFITS	HOW TO IMPLEMENT

New Recipes	Keeps meals exciting	Experiment with a new healthy recipe each week
Different Exercises	Engages various muscle groups	Try yoga, swimming, or hiking in addition to routine workouts
Stress-Relief	Mental clarity and emotional balance	Add meditation, journaling, or listening to music daily

wellness through reliable sources. When you're well-informed, you're better equipped to make decisions that align with your long-term health objectives.

Reflect on your journey regularly. Set aside time each month to review your journal entries and assess how you've handled setbacks and achieved goals. This periodic reflection helps reinforce what's working and allows you to adjust strategies that could be improved.

Lastly, practice patience and persistence. Long-term health is not achieved overnight; it's the cumulative effect of consistent, day-to-day effort. Trust the process, stay motivated, and remember that every step you take towards better health is significant.

Tools and Resources for Tracking Progress and Staying Committed

As we navigate this cleansing path, it's crucial to track our progress and stay committed to the regimen. So, let's delve into some effective tools and resources that can help us achieve this.

1. **Tracking Progress**: Keeping a journal has been incredibly beneficial. By writing down daily experiences, symptoms, meals, and emotional states, I can pinpoint what works best for my body. This journal becomes a personal health diary that reflects both the successes and struggles. It tells me when I'm progressing and alerts me when I might need to tweak something.

Another valuable tool is a digital tracker or app. There are numerous health tracking apps available that allow us to log food intake, water consumption, physical activities, and even moods. Apps like MyFitnessPal or Cronometer provide nutritional breakdowns of meals and help keep tabs on daily nutrient intake. This data can be crucial for aligning with Dr. Sebi's alkaline diet principles.

For those who prefer visuals over numbers, progress photos are excellent motivators. Taking weekly photos provides a visual testament to our body's transformation over time. Comparing these pictures can be encouraging and often showcases changes that the scale may not reflect.

2. **Staying Committed**: Commitment is arguably one of the most challenging aspects of any health journey. Setting clear goals from the outset is indispensable. Goals should be specific, measurable, achievable, relevant, and time-bound (SMART). Setting such structured objectives helps in maintaining focus and provides clear milestones to celebrate along the way.

Community support also plays an integral role in staying committed. Joining online forums or local groups of people who follow Dr. Sebi's teachings can provide emotional support as well as practical advice. Being part of a community fosters a sense of belonging and provides a platform to share experiences, recipes, challenges, and triumphs.

Accountability partners are another fantastic resource for commitment. Whether it's a friend, family member, or someone from an online group, having someone else aware of your goals helps keep you on track. Checking in regularly with an accountability partner ensures you remain committed even during tough times.

Tools & Equipment

TOOL	PURPOSE	NOTES
Journal	Logging daily experiences	Opt for one with sections for food intake and symptoms
Health Apps	Tracking nutrients and activities	MyFitnessPal, Cronometer
Progress Photos	Visual tracking	Take once per week at same time
Blender	Smoothie preparation	Ensures smooth integration of fruits/vegetables
Water Bottle	Hydration tracking	Makes sure you meet daily water goals

Let's not forget about meal prepping supplies too – containers for portion control, cooking utensils specifically for making Sebi-approved meals, etc., will streamline meal preparations ensuring we don't stray away from our diet. Schedule regular health check-ins with your healthcare provider if you have specific medical conditions or concerns related to this diet.

CHAPTER 8

Maintenance and Avanced Strategies

Guidelines for Continuing Health Improvements After the Initial Cleanse

As we move beyond the initial cleanse, it's important to understand that maintaining our health and continuing the positive trajectory we started requires dedication, discipline, and knowledge. I want to share some practical guidelines that will help you not just preserve but further enhance your well-being.

1. **Adopt a Nutrient-Rich Diet**: After completing the mucus cleanse, our bodies are in an optimal state to absorb nutrients. It's crucial to maintain a diet rich in fresh fruits, vegetables, whole grains, nuts, seeds, and legumes. These foods provide essential vitamins, minerals, and antioxidants that support overall health.

   ➢ Prefer organic produce to avoid pesticides.
   ➢ Focus on consuming a variety of colorful fruits and vegetables.
   ➢ Use herbs like ginger, turmeric, and garlic which have anti-inflammatory properties.

2. **Stay Hydrated**: Water is key to almost every bodily function. Aim to drink at least 8-10 glasses of water daily. You can also include herbal teas and fresh vegetable juices as part of your hydration routine.

3. **Regular Exercise**: Incorporate physical activity into your daily routine. Exercise helps in maintaining a healthy weight, reduces stress levels, and improves cardiovascular health. Even simple activities like walking, stretching or yoga can make a big difference.

4. **Mindful Eating Practices**: Slow down and savor your meals. Chew thoroughly to aid digestion and absorption of nutrients. Avoid overeating by listening to your body's hunger signals and stopping when you feel satisfied.

5. **Regular Detoxification**: Even after the initial cleanse, it's beneficial to incorporate periodic mini-detoxes into your lifestyle. This could be in the form of fasting, intermittent fasting or simply having a day dedicated to raw fruits and vegetables every week.

6. **Adequate Sleep**: Ensuring you get enough quality rest is pivotal for overall health. Aim for 7-9 hours of sleep per night. Keep a regular sleep schedule by going to bed and waking up at the same time each day.

7. **Stress Management**: Stress can negatively impact our health in myriad ways. Techniques such as meditation, deep breathing exercises, spending time in nature, or engaging in hobbies can help manage stress effectively.

8. **Avoid Toxic Substances**: Steer clear of processed foods, refined sugars, alcohol, tobacco and other harmful substances that can reintroduce toxins into your system.

9. **Support System**: Surround yourself with supportive people who understand your health goals and encourage you along the way. Joining health communities or groups can also offer shared learning experiences and motivation.

SUGGESTED WEEKLY ROUTINE POST-CLEANSE		
DAY	ACTIVITY	NOTES
MON	Light Exercise (Yoga/Walk)	Aim for 30 mins
TUE	Hydration Focus	Drink herbal tea in addition to water
WED	Raw Food Day	Consume only raw fruits & veggies
THU	Mindfulness Practice	Start meditation or breathing exercises
FRI	Nutrient-Rich Meals	Ensure diverse intake from all food groups
SAT	Leisure & Relaxation	Engage in a hobby or nature walk
SUN	Adequate Rest	Plan for an early bedtime

Stay informed about nutrition and health developments by reading books like *"Dr. Sebi Mucus Cleanse Bible"* and following reputable sources. Continuous learning empowers you to make better health choices. Let's remember that health is a journey, not a destination. This path requires ongoing commitment and a willingness to adjust based on how our bodies respond to different practices and foods.

Advanced Detox and Mucus Removal Strategies

Having detailed the basics of cleansing, it's time to explore advanced strategies to target mucus buildup and achieve optimal health. While the initial cleansing steps lay the groundwork, advancing your detox can help eliminate hidden mucus deposits, toxins and enhance your overall well-being.

Integrating More Alkaline Foods

My first recommendation is to bolster our diet with a wider variety of alkaline foods. A highly alkaline diet disrupts the acidic environment that causes mucus buildup. Fruits like berries, cherries, and melons are excellent choices. Also, vegetables such as leafy greens, cucumbers, and bell peppers should be part of daily meals. Remember to keep processed foods, meat, dairy, and refined sugars out of your diet—they're significant contributors to acidity and mucus formation.

Herbal Remedies

Certain herbs have shown profound effects on detoxification and mucus dissolution:

1. **Burdock Root:** Known for its blood-purifying properties. It supports liver function and aids in removing toxins.
2. **Bladderwrack:** Rich in iodine which boosts thyroid function and maintains hormonal balance.
3. **Sarsaparilla:** Known for its anti-inflammatory properties; this herb helps in flushing out toxins through increased urine output.
4. **Yellow Dock:** A potent herb that enhances digestive health, tackling constipation which may contribute to mucus buildup.

Fasting Methods

Beyond intermittent fasting mentioned earlier, extended fasting periods can take cleansing to the next level:

1. **24-Hour Dry Fast:** This entails abstaining from both food and water for a complete day. It gives your digestive system a break, allowing it to remove any latent waste more efficiently.
2. **Juice Fasting:** Consuming only vegetable and fruit juices for several days provides essential nutrients while keeping caloric intake low—facilitating an intensive cleanse.

In my experience, especially for those new to fasting or with underlying health conditions, it's critical to consult a healthcare professional beforehand.

Sweating it Out

Frequent sauna sessions or steam baths are effective ways of mobilizing accumulated toxins stored in fatty tissues. Perspiration during these heat therapies brings these toxins to the skin's surface where they can be washed away. Aim for sessions lasting 20-30 mins at least three times weekly.

Lymphatic System Support

Our lymphatic system plays a pivotal role in detoxification by transporting waste materials away from tissues into the bloodstream. Here's how we can give it a helpful nudge:

1. **Rebounding:** Jumping on a mini-trampoline stimulates lymphatic fluid circulation.
2. **Dry Brushing:** Gently brushing skin towards the heart using natural bristle brushes helps move lymphatic fluid along.

Customized Dietary Plans

Over time I've realized that one size doesn't fit all when it comes to dietary changes required for detoxifying effectively:

1. **Individual Assessments:** Track symptoms and energy levels daily in a journal.
2. **Personalized Adjustments:** Modify your intake of certain foods based on observations—adding or reducing particular items.

For example: If mucosal build-up seems persistent despite dietary changes, consider further reducing starchy vegetables or grains.

Oxygenation Techniques

Proper oxygenation is another pivotal element in advanced detox and mucus removal strategies. Oxygen is essential for cellular health, energy production, and effective detoxification. Here are some methods to enhance oxygenation in your body:

1. **Deep Breathing Exercises:** Practice deep breathing exercises daily. Inhale deeply through your nose, allowing your diaphragm to expand, and exhale slowly through your mouth. This not only increases oxygen intake but also promotes relaxation.
2. **Physical Activities:** Engage in regular physical activities such as brisk walking, jogging, or swimming. These activities not only improve cardiovascular health but also boost oxygen levels in the blood.

3. **Pranayama:** This ancient practice from yoga involves specific breathing techniques that enhance lung capacity and oxygen intake. Simple techniques like alternate nostril breathing can be highly effective.

Integrating these oxygenation techniques into your daily routine can significantly support your ongoing detox efforts by ensuring that your cells receive the oxygen they need to function optimally and expel toxins effectively.

Long-term Health Plans Incorporating Dr. Sebi's Teachings

When most people think of Dr. Sebi, they often focus on his various cleanses and fasting methods that help to eliminate mucus and impurities from the body. While these cleansing periods are indeed powerful tools for detoxification, the real magic lies in the long-term health plans that can transform your life long after a cleanse is completed.

It's clear that one must maintain a diet rich in alkaline foods to ensure that the body remains free from excess mucus and toxins. Following Dr. Sebi's nutritional guide is pivotal here. He recommends a diet consisting primarily of raw fruits and vegetables, nuts, seeds, and grains that are naturally alkaline. This isn't about temporary dietary adjustments; rather, it is a permanent lifestyle change aimed at achieving optimum health.

An essential aspect of this long-term health plan is proper hydration. Drinking spring water or water with added natural minerals helps maintain an alkaline environment within the body. Aim to drink at least 3 liters of water each day. This improves not just digestion but also overall cellular functions.

For protein sources, Dr. Sebi advises incorporating plant-based options such as quinoa, hemp seeds, chia seeds, and legumes like chickpeas and lentils into your meals regularly. These foods offer sufficient protein without compromising on alkalinity.

Here is a quick guide for daily consumption based on Dr. Sebi's recommendations:

CATEGORY	DAILY SERVINGS
Fruits	3-4 servings (e.g., berries, mangoes)
Vegetables	5-6 servings (e.g., kale, cucumbers)
Nuts/Seeds	1-2 servings (e.g., walnuts, chia seeds)

Grains	2-3 servings (e.g., quinoa, wild rice)
Legumes	1-2 servings (e.g., lentils, chickpeas)
Water	At least 3 liters

Exercise is another critical component of maintaining long-term health as per Dr. Sebi's teachings. Regular physical activity stimulates the lymphatic system and aids in ongoing detoxification processes. Activities such as yoga, walking, or even light jogging can be integrated into your weekly routine for best results.

Herbal supplements also play a key role in supporting sustained wellness. Herbs like Burdock root for blood purification, Bladderwrack for iodine supply and sea moss for mineral replenishment should be incorporated into daily routines to promote optimal bodily functions.

Mental wellness cannot be overlooked either in this holistic approach to health promoted by Dr. Sebi. Consistent practices such as meditation or mindfulness exercises can significantly reduce stress levels and improve mental clarity over time.

Routine medical check-ups should also be part of your long-term plan to track progress and adapt strategies as needed.

To sustain energy levels throughout the day, focus on having balanced meals and take short breaks to rest when needed. Personally, I've found that including small snacks such as fresh fruit or a handful of nuts can keep my energy stable.

SNACK IDEAS	NUTRITION BENEFIT
Almonds	Rich in healthy fats and protein
Apples	High in fiber for steady energy
Carrot sticks	Provide vitamins and minerals
Smoothies	Easy way to pack in fruits and greens

Remember, it's crucial to listen to your body. If you're feeling run down, make sure you're getting enough sleep and managing stress effectively. Meditation, mindfulness practices, or simply spending time in nature can make a big difference.

Adopting Dr. Sebi's teachings into a long-term health plan involves more than just diet and exercise—it's about creating a balanced lifestyle. This holistic approach aims for overall well-being, ensuring that we not only live longer but with vitality.

With dedication to these principles, I'm confident you will witness amazing transformations in your health and life.

CHAPTER 9

Frequently Asked Questions

Addressing Common Questions and Concerns

Now, I want to take a moment to address some of the most common questions and concerns people have about these methods. Understanding these aspects can make the journey smoother and more rewarding.

1. Why Alkaline Foods?

One of the first questions that often arises is why Dr. Sebi emphasizes the consumption of alkaline foods. The answer lies in the belief that an alkaline diet helps cleanse and restore the body to its optimal health state. By maintaining an alkaline internal environment, it's thought that one can reduce mucus buildup and foster an environment less conducive to disease.

2. Can I Eat Any Fruit or Vegetable?

Not necessarily. Dr. Sebi's nutritional guide specifies particular fruits, vegetables, grains, nuts, seeds, and oils that are believed to be most beneficial in preventing mucus accumulation in the body. For example, fruits like apples and grapes are encouraged while avoiding hybrid or genetically modified organisms (GMO) fruits like seedless watermelon.

3. How Long Should I Follow the Cleanse?

The duration can vary depending on personal goals and health conditions. Some people may choose to follow the cleanse for a few weeks, while others might adhere to it for several months or even adopt it as a long-term lifestyle change. It's crucial to listen to your body and consult with a healthcare provider before making any drastic changes.

4. Will I Experience Detox Symptoms?

Many people experience detox symptoms when they start the cleanse because their body begins to expel toxins stored in tissues. These symptoms might include headaches, fatigue, or flu-like symptoms; however, they are generally temporary.

5. Is It Safe for Everyone?

While many have found success with Dr. Sebi's methods, it's essential to remember that everyone's body is different. If you have underlying health issues or are pregnant or nursing, consultation with a healthcare professional is strongly advised before undertaking any new dietary regimen.

6. What If I Slip Up?

Consistency is key, but occasional lapses happen to everyone from time to time. If you slip up, don't be hard on yourself; get back on track as soon as possible. Remember that this is a journey towards better health rather than perfection.

7. Are There Specific Supplements I Should Take?

Dr. Sebi recommended certain natural supplements derived from herbs like burdock root, bladderwrack, and sea moss due to their high mineral content which supports overall immunity and detoxification processes.

8. Can I Maintain My Energy Levels During This Cleanse?

Yes! Many people worry they will feel weak or tired while cleansing, but you can maintain your energy by consuming nutrient-dense foods that are low in acidity but high in minerals like leafy greens, fresh fruit juices, and herbal teas.

9. Why No Animal Products?

Animal products are often acid-forming which means they could contribute to mucus formation within the body according to Dr. Sebi's methodology. Eliminating them from your diet is believed to help maintain an alkaline state which supports overall wellness.

10. How Do I Handle Social Situations?

Navigating social settings while following Dr. Sebi's cleanse can be challenging, but with some planning, it's manageable. Inform your friends and family about your dietary choices ahead of time so they can accommodate you or at least be aware. Bring your own dishes to gatherings if possible; this ensures that there will be something you can eat. When dining out, research restaurants that offer menu items aligned with the nutritional guide or request modifications to suit your needs.

11. Will I Lose Weight?

Weight loss is a common outcome of the cleanse due to the dietary restrictions and emphasis on natural, whole foods. Many people find they shed excess pounds as their bodies expel toxins and switch to a cleaner diet. However, the primary goal is improved health and well-being rather than weight loss alone.

12. What About Exercise?

Incorporating moderate exercise can complement the cleanse by promoting better circulation and aiding in toxin elimination through sweat. Activities such as walking, yoga, or light cardio are recommended. Always listen to your body and avoid strenuous workouts if you feel fatigued.

13. Can I Drink Alcohol or Coffee?

Alcohol and coffee are generally discouraged during the cleanse due to their acid-forming properties and potential to stimulate mucus production. Opt for herbal teas or water infused with fruit instead.

14. How Can I Ensure Proper Nutrition?

Following Dr. Sebi's nutritional guide should provide most essential nutrients needed for optimal health. Including a wide variety of approved foods ensures you get a range of vitamins and minerals. If you have specific concerns about nutrient deficiencies, consulting with a healthcare provider might be beneficial.

15. Can I Customize My Cleanse?

Absolutely! Dr. Sebi's principles offer flexibility for personalization based on your specific needs and preferences within his recommended guidelines. Tailoring meals according to what sustains you best can make it easier to stick to the regimen long term.

By addressing these common questions and concerns, my goal is to provide clarity and support as you embark on your journey toward better health through Dr. Sebi's mucus cleanse methods. Remember, dedication and consistency are key – but always personalize your approach based on how your body reacts and feels throughout the process.

Additional Advice on Herbal Supplements and Dietary Adjustments

When following Dr. Sebi's recommendations for minimizing mucus accumulation in the body, one must delve deeper into the wealth of herbal supplements available and make thoughtful dietary adjustments. From my experience, these additional steps have been highly effective in achieving a full-body cleanse and promoting overall well-being.

1. **Herbal Supplements:** Beyond the core herbs discussed previously, several other herbal supplements can offer substantial benefits. These herbs complement Dr. Sebi's foundational approach and bring additional advantages to the table.

   a) *Irish Moss:* Rich in essential minerals, Irish moss is great for soothing mucus membranes and improving respiratory health. It's also superb for skin health due to its high vitamin and mineral content.

   b) *Chaparral:* Known for its potent antioxidants, chaparral can detoxify the body at a cellular level. It's also helpful in alleviating respiratory issues by breaking down mucus.

   c) *Red Clover:* This plant is an excellent blood purifier and aids in removing toxins that contribute to mucus buildup. Additionally, it supports lung function.

   d) *Licorice Root:* Licorice root has anti-inflammatory properties that soothe irritated mucus membranes, particularly in the throat and lungs.

   e) *Blue Vervain:* This herb acts as a natural expectorant, which helps to thin mucus, making it easier for your body to eliminate it.

2. **Dietary Adjustments:** Making appropriate dietary changes will further reap the benefits of using herbal supplements to reduce mucus production.

   a) *Increase Water Intake:* Regular hydration supports all bodily functions but is crucial for flushing out toxins that contribute to mucus production.

   b) *Fermented Foods:* Foods such as sauerkraut, kimchi, and kombucha introduce beneficial bacteria into your gut, enhancing digestion and reducing inflammation that leads to excess mucus.

   c) *Limit Dairy Products:* Dairy can often increase mucus production. Switching to plant-based alternatives such as almond milk or oat milk can make a significant difference.

   d) *Avoid Refined Sugars:* High sugar intake contributes to inflammation and should be minimized. Opt for natural sweeteners like honey or maple syrup.

   e) *Whole Grains:* Brown rice, quinoa, and oats are preferable choices over refined grains since they are less likely to produce excess mucus.

f) *Spices like Ginger and Turmeric*: Both of these have excellent anti-inflammatory properties which may assist in reducing mucus production.

HYDRATING FOODS CHART		
FOOD	**WATER CONTENT (%)**	**BENEFITS**
Cucumber	95%	Hydrates and flushes out toxins
Watermelon	92%	High water content; helps clear out excess fluids
Zucchini	95%	Promotes hydration; assists digestion
Strawberries	91%	Packed with vitamins; supports immune function

Understanding how different herbs and dietary changes contribute to reducing mucus can provide you with powerful tools on your journey towards better health. By incorporating these additional herbal supplements and making mindful dietary adjustments, you align yourself more closely with Dr. Sebi's philosophy of natural wellness, creating an environment within your body where health can flourish naturally.

Remember always to consult with a healthcare provider before making any major changes to your diet or supplement regimen, especially if you have existing health conditions or take medication regularly.

Clarifications on Misconceptions About the Alkaline Diet and Herbal Health

I've encountered many misconceptions about the alkaline diet over the years. It's time to set the record straight and provide clear, factual information. Many people believe that switching to an alkaline diet is a quick fix for every health issue, but it's important to understand its true benefits and limitations.

Misconception 1: The Alkaline Diet Can Cure All Diseases

One of the prevailing myths is that the alkaline diet is a cure-all for every disease. While I'm a strong proponent of the benefits tied to an alkaline lifestyle, it's important to understand its limitations and context. An alkaline diet focuses on consuming foods that have an alkalizing effect on the body. This includes a diet rich in fruits and vegetables while limiting processed foods, meat, and dairy.

While an improved diet can certainly contribute to better health outcomes and potentially reduce certain disease risks, it should not be considered a singular solution. Always consult healthcare professionals for medical conditions that require specific treatments.

Misconception 2: pH Levels Can Be Radically Altered by Diet Alone

Another common misunderstanding is that you can significantly change your body's pH level solely through what you eat. It's a fact that while food influences your body's pH levels somewhat, your body regulates pH levels very tightly, maintaining blood pH between 7.35 and 7.45 regardless of dietary intake.

What you eat can impact your urine's pH level but not drastically change your blood's pH level because the body has sophisticated mechanisms to maintain this balance. However, an alkaline diet does promote overall health benefits due to nutrient-rich food choices. These foods help foster a healthier internal environment that supports systems like digestion, detoxification, and inflammation reduction.

Misconception 3: All Herbs are Created Equal

Not all herbs are beneficial or work universally for everyone; this is an area where many misconceptions reside. The appropriateness of any herb can depend on one's individual health situation, existing medical conditions, medications taken, and even genetic makeup.

For instance, while Dr. Sebi recommended using burdock root for its blood-purifying properties or sarsaparilla for its high iron content among other benefits—individual responses can vary greatly. To simplify this point:

HERB	PRIMARY BENEFIT	POTENTIAL CONSIDERATIONS
Burdock Root	Blood purification; detoxification	May cause allergic reactions in some individuals
Sarsaparilla	High iron content; inflammation reduction	Ensure no incompatibility with medications
Elderberry	Immune system boost	Overuse can cause digestive issues
Dandelion	Supports liver health; acts as diuretic	Excessive use may cause electrolyte imbalances

It's crucial always to consult with knowledgeable healthcare providers when incorporating herbal remedies into your health regime, especially if you are on medication or have pre-existing conditions.

Misconception 4: Immediate Results From Diet Changes

Many expect immediate results when shifting to an alkaline diet or integrating herbs into their lifestyle. However, bodily systems need time to adjust before noticeable changes take effect. Patience is paramount when making dietary adjustments for long-term wellness.

Tasks like reducing processed food intake, incorporating more vegetables, and staying hydrated responsibly contribute to a gradual improvement in health. The idea is to create enduring habits that foster wellness over time instead of expecting an overnight transformation.

Misconception 5: Alkaline Diet and Cancer Cure

Another significant misconception is that the alkaline diet can cure cancer directly. While it's true that an alkaline diet can promote a healthier body environment, there is no credible scientific evidence suggesting it can cure cancer. This misinformation can be dangerous as it may lead individuals to forego conventional treatments proven to be effective. Consultation with oncologists and healthcare providers remains essential for anyone dealing with cancer.

Misconception 6: All Alkaline Foods Are Suitable for Everyone

Not all alkaline foods will benefit everyone in the same way. Individual needs vary, especially for those with specific health conditions such as kidney disease or digestive issues. For instance, although citrus fruits like lemons and limes are considered alkaline-forming, excessive consumption could aggravate symptoms for people with acid reflux or gastritis. Listening to your body and consulting healthcare professionals helps tailor the diet to your specific needs.

An alkaline diet has numerous advantages, including its nutrient-rich composition and potential health benefits, but it should be adopted as part of a broader strategy for well-being. Always seek advice from knowledgeable healthcare providers when making significant dietary changes or incorporating herbal remedies into your routine. Consistency, patience, and professional guidance are key components of achieving genuine lasting health improvements.

CONCLUSION

As I reflect on the journey outlined in the "Dr. Sebi Mucus Cleanse Bible," it's clear that the path to optimal health requires dedication and a shift in lifestyle. Dr. Sebi's philosophy revolves around the importance of removing excess mucus from the body, which, according to him, is a major contributor to many health issues. By embracing a plant-based diet rich in alkaline foods and specific herbs, we can effectively cleanse our bodies and restore balance.

Throughout this book, we learned that mucus can become problematic when it accumulates excessively due to poor diet and environmental factors. This buildup can lead to conditions such as chronic sinusitis or bronchitis, as evidenced by Susan's and Mark's case studies. The connection between excess mucus and common diseases has been clearly established, reinforcing the necessity of a thorough detoxification process.

Dr. Sebi's methods are backed by both traditional practices and scientific insights. His recommended herbs and foods, such as sea moss and burdock root, have been shown to aid in cleansing and supporting the body's natural detox pathways, like the liver, kidneys, lungs, and skin. Preparing for this cleanse involves not only adopting new dietary habits but also mental readiness. It's crucial to address fears and set realistic goals to ensure a smooth transition into this new lifestyle.

The structured 28-day detox plan is comprehensive, guiding us through phases of transition, deep cleansing, fasting, resetting, reintroduction of foods, and maintenance. Each phase plays a role in systematically reducing mucus while promoting overall wellness. The detailed meal plans and recipes included provide practical ways to incorporate these nutritional guidelines into everyday life.

Integrating these principles beyond the initial cleanse is essential for long-term health benefits. Strategies for dining out, traveling, and family adaptation ensure that Dr. Sebi's methods are sustainable in various aspects of life. Overcoming challenges is part of the process; practical solutions are offered to handle setbacks and maintain progress.

"Dr. Sebi Mucus Cleanse Bible" empowers us with knowledge and tools necessary for a healthier life free from excess mucus related complications. By following Dr. Sebi's holistic approach with commitment and openness to change, we pave the way for lasting health improvements that go beyond mere symptom relief; we achieve true wellness by fostering an internal environment where disease cannot thrive.

Get Your <u>Free</u> Bonuses Now

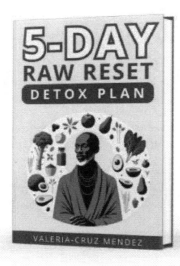 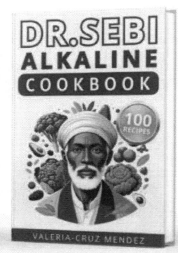 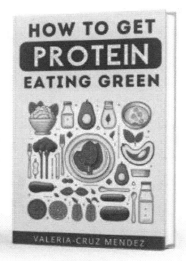

BONUS #1: 5-Day Raw Reset Detox Plan

Jumpstart your journey to wellness with **a 5-day detox plan** designed to cleanse your body, reset your system, and boost your energy levels, all while staying true to Dr. Sebi's principles.

BONUS #2: Dr. Sebi Alkaline Cookbook

Delve into over **100 mouth-watering alkaline recipes** that not only adhere to the alkaline diet but also turn every meal into a healing, nutritious feast for your body.

BONUS #3: How to Get Protein Eating Green

Discover the secrets of **meeting your protein needs with plant-based sources**, ensuring your nutrition is holistic, sustainable, and perfectly aligned with an alkaline lifestyle.

Scan with your phone's camera **OR** go to:

https://shorturl.at/gjpy8

Made in United States
Orlando, FL
07 October 2024